I0428376

1 Where Did Ebola Come From?

In some parts of Africa, myths that Ebola was brought to the regions by health care workers have hurt the ability of workers to respond to the outbreak. But where did Ebola really come from?

The true reservoir for Ebola — that is, where the virus hides when it's not causing outbreaks in people — is not known for sure, but experts say that bats are the likely source of the deadly virus. "There's a strong circumstantial case, but we haven't actually got a total smoking gun," said Derek Gatherer, a bioinformatics researcher at Lancaster University in the United Kingdom.

The first known human cases of Ebola occurred in 1976 during two simultaneous outbreaks in Sudan and the Democratic Republic of Congo, which sickened more than 600 people, according to the World Health Organization.

Nearly 20 years later, in 2005, researchers looking for the reservoir of Ebola sampled more than 1,000 small animals in the Central African nations of Gabon and the Republic of the Congo, which have also experienced outbreaks of Ebola. They tested 679 bats, 222 birds and 129 small terrestrial vertebrates.

The only animals found to harbor the Ebola virus were bats, specifically, three species of fruit bat: The hammer-headed bat, Franquet's epauletted fruit bat, and the little collared fruit bat.

At least two of these fruit bat species are also found in Guinea — which is where the current Ebola outbreak in West Africa began — so it's possible that these bats were sources for the outbreak, Gatherer told Live Science.

Researchers in Guinea are now sampling bats in that region to see if any test positive for Ebola, Gatherer said. The current outbreak has sickened more than 10,000 people, and of these, more than 4,500 people have died, according to the World Health Organization.

If bats are the source of the virus, one way people might become infected is by handling bats that are eaten for food, Gatherer said. For example, bat soup is a delicacy in the region.

Officials in Guinea took the step of banning the consumption and sale of bats in March, after the outbreak began, he said.

But it's not necessarily the eating itself that leads to Ebola infection —cooking would likely kill the virus, Gatherer said. Instead, it's the butchering of bats and handling of raw bat meat that's more risky, he said.

Still, it's not known for certain whether bats are the only reservoirs of the virus, or whether it is infections in bats that spilled over to people, Gatherer said.

A stronger case could be made for bats as the source of infection if researchers found the same genetic sequence for Ebola in people and in bats in the region, Gatherer said.

There is some evidence that, rather than being a virus that is always carried by bats, Ebola is actually causing an outbreak in bats — that is, it is being spread among bat populations.

By looking at the virus' genetic material, researchers have found that the same Ebola virus has been carried from bats in Central Africa to bats in West Africa over the past 10 years, Gatherer said.

The virus could have been carried by bats or by people, but if it was carried by people, researchers would have expected to see cases along the way, Gatherer said. "It's probably more likely that there's an epidemic going on in bats, but we can't be absolutely certain," Gatherer said.

Who Discovered Ebola In The Virus Detective 1976

Nearly 40 years ago, a young Belgian scientist travelled to a remote part of the Congolese rainforest - his task was to help find out why so many people were dying from an unknown and terrifying disease.

In September 1976, a package containing a shiny, blue thermos flask arrived at the Institute of Tropical Medicine in Antwerp, Belgium.

Working in the lab that day was Peter Piot, a 27-year-old scientist and medical school graduate training as a clinical microbiologist.

"It was just a normal flask like any other you would use to keep coffee warm," recalls Piot, now Director of the London School of Hygiene and Tropical Medicine.

But this thermos wasn't carrying coffee - inside was an altogether different cargo. Nestled amongst a few melting ice cubes were vials of blood along with a note.

It was from a Belgian doctor based in what was then Zaire, now the Democratic Republic of Congo - his handwritten message explained that the blood was that of a nun, also from Belgium, who had fallen ill with a mysterious illness which he couldn't identify.

This unusual delivery had travelled all the way from Zaire's capital city Kinshasa, on a commercial flight, in one of the passengers' hand luggage.

"When we opened the thermos, we saw that one of the vials was broken and blood was mixing with the water from the melted ice," says Piot.

He and his colleagues were unaware just how dangerous that was. As the blood leaked into the icy water so too did a deadly unknown virus.

The samples were treated like numerous others the lab had tested before, but when the scientists placed some of the cells under an electron microscope they saw something they didn't expect.

"We saw a gigantic worm like structure - gigantic by viral standards," says Piot. "It's a very unusual shape for a virus, only one other virus looked like that and that was the Marburg virus."

The Marburg virus was first recognised in 1967 when 31 people became ill with haemorrhagic fever in the cities of Marburg and Frankfurt in Germany and in Belgrade, the capital of Yugoslavia. This Marburg outbreak was associated with laboratory staff who were working with infected monkeys imported from Uganda - seven people died.

Piot knew how serious Marburg could be - but after consulting experts around the world he got confirmation that what he was seeing under the microscope wasn't Marburg - this was something else, something never seen before.

"It's hard to describe but the main emotion I had was one of real, incredible excitement," says Piot. "There was a feeling of being very privileged, that this was a moment of discovery."

News had reached Antwerp that the nun, who was under the care of the doctor in Zaire, had died. The team also learnt that many others were falling ill with this mysterious illness in a remote area in the north of the country - their symptoms include fever, diarrhoea and vomiting followed by bleeding and eventually death.

Two weeks later Piot, who had never been to Africa before, was on a flight to Kinshasa. "It was an overnight flight and I couldn't sleep. I was so excited about seeing Africa for the first time, about investigating this new virus and about stopping the epidemic."

The journey didn't end in Kinshasa - the team had to travel to the centre of the outbreak, a village in the equatorial rainforest, about 1,000km (620 miles) further north.

"The personal physician of President Mobutu, the leader of Zaire at that time, arranged a C-130 transport aircraft for us," recalls Piot. They loaded a Landrover, fuel and all the equipment they needed on to the plane.

When the C-130 landed in Bumba, a river port situated on the northernmost point of the Congo River, the fear surrounding the mysterious disease was tangible. Even the pilots didn't want to hang around for long - they kept the airplane's engines running as the team unloaded their kit.

"As they left they shouted 'Adieu,'" says Piot. "In French, people say 'Au Revoir' to say 'See you again', but when they say 'Adieu' - well, that's like saying, 'We'll never see you again.'"

Standing on the tarmac watching the plane leave, facing a deadly unknown virus in an unfamiliar place, some people might have regretted the decision to go there.

"I wasn't scared. The excitement of discovery and wanting to stop the epidemic was driving everything. We heard far more people were dying from the disease than we originally thought and we wanted to get to work," Piot says. The curiosity and sense of adventure that brought Piot to this point had been ignited many years earlier when he was a young boy growing up in a small rural village in the Flanders region of Belgium.

A museum near Piot's home was dedicated to a local saint who worked with leprosy patients, and it was here that he got his first glimpse into the world of disease and microbiology.

"I decided one day to cycle to the museum. The old pictures I saw there of those suffering from leprosy fascinated me," he says. "That sparked my interest in medicine - it gave me a thirst for scientific knowledge, a desire to help people and I hoped it would give me a passport to the world."

It did give Piot a passport to the world. The team's final destination was the village of Yambuku - about 120km (75 miles) from Bumba, where the plane had left them.

Yambuku was home to an old Catholic mission - it had a hospital and a school run by a priest and nuns, all of them from Belgium.

"The area was beautiful. The mission was surrounded by lush rainforest and the earth was red - the nature was incredibly rich but the people were so poor," says Piot. "Joseph Conrad called that place 'The Heart of Darkness', but I thought there was a lot of light there."

The beauty of Yambuku belied the horror that was unfolding for the people that lived there.

When Piot arrived, the first people he met were a group of nuns and a priest who had retreated to a guesthouse and established their own cordon sanitaire - a barrier used to prevent the spread of disease.

There was a sign on the cord, written in the local Lingala language that read, "Please stop, anybody who crosses here may die."

"They had already lost four of their colleagues to the disease," says Piot. "They were praying and waiting for death."

Piot jumped over the cordon and told them that the team would help them and stop the epidemic. "When you are 27, you have all this confidence," he says.

The nuns told the newly arrived scientists what had happened, they spoke about their colleagues and those in the village who had died and how they tried to help as best they could.

The priority was to stop the epidemic, but first the team needed to find out how this virus was moving from person to person - by air, in food, by direct contact or spread by insects. "We had to start asking questions. It was really like a detective story," says Piot.

To investigate the spread of the virus the team drew maps and plotted each village they visited

These were the three questions they asked:

• How did the epidemic evolve? Knowing when each person caught the virus gave clues to what kind of infection this was - from here the story of the virus began to emerge.

• Where did the infected people come from? The team visited all the surrounding villages and mapped out the number of infections - it was clear that the outbreak was closely related to areas served by the local hospital.

• Who gets infected? The team found that more women than men caught the disease and particularly women between 18 and 30 years old - it turned out that many of the women in this age group were pregnant and many had attended an antenatal clinic at the hospital.

The mystery of the virus was beginning to unravel.

The team then discovered that the women who attended the antenatal clinic all received a routine injection. Each morning, just five syringes would be distributed, the needles would be reused and so the virus was spread between the patients.

"That's how we began to figure it out," recalls Piot. "You do it by talking, looking at the statistics and using logical deduction."

The team also noticed that people were getting ill after attending funerals. When someone dies from Ebola, the body is full of the virus - any direct contact, such as washing or preparation of the deceased without protection can be a serious risk.

The next step was to stop the transmission of the virus.

"We systematically went from village to village and if someone was ill they would be put into quarantine," says Piot. "We would also quarantine anyone in direct contact with those infected and we would ensure everyone knew how to correctly bury those who had died from the virus."

The closure of the hospital, the use of quarantine and making sure the community had all the necessary information eventually brought an end to the epidemic - but nearly 300 people died.

Piot and his colleagues had learned a lot about the virus during three months in Yambuku, but it still lacked a name.

"We didn't want to name it after the village, Yambuku, because it's so stigmatising. You don't want to be associated with that," says Piot.

The team decided to name the virus after a river. They had a map of Zaire, although not a very detailed one, and the closest river they could see was the Ebola River. From that point on, the virus that arrived in a flask in Antwerp all those months earlier would be known as the Ebola virus.

In February 2014, Piot returned to Yambuku for only the second time since 1976, to mark his 65th birthday. He met Sukato Mandzomba, one of the few who caught the virus in 1976 and survived. "It was fantastic to meet him again, it was a very moving moment," says Piot.

Back then, Mandzomba was a nurse in the local hospital and could speak French so the pair had managed to build up a rapport. "He's still living in Yambuku and still working in the hospital - he's now running the lab there and it's impeccable. I was really impressed," Piot says.

It's 38 years since that initial outbreak and the world is now experiencing its worst Ebola epidemic ever. So far more than 4,500 people have died. The current situation has been called unprecedented, the spread of the disease across three countries making it more complicated to deal with than ever before.

In the absence of any vaccine or cure, the advice for this outbreak is much the same as it was in the 1970s. "Soap, gloves, isolating patients, not reusing needles and quarantining the contacts of those who are ill - in theory it should be very easy to contain Ebola," says Piot.

In practice though, other factors can make fighting an Ebola outbreak a difficult task. People who become ill and their families may be stigmatised by the community - resulting in a reluctance to come forward for help. Cultural beliefs lead some to think the disease is caused by witchcraft, while others are hostile towards health workers.

"We shouldn't forget that this is a disease of poverty, of dysfunctional health systems - and of distrust," says Piot.

For this reason, information, communication and involvement of community leaders are as important as the classical medical approach, he argues.

Ebola changed Piot's life - following the discovery of the virus, he went on to research the Aids epidemic in Africa and became the founding executive director of the UNAIDS organisation.

"It led me to do things I thought only happened in books. It gave me a mission in life to work on health in developing countries," he says.

"It was not only the discovery of a virus but also of myself."

Ebola's Murderous Path From A Toddler To Global Mayhem

Geneva (AFP) - When a toddler in a remote Guinean village suddenly died from a mysterious fever last December, no one could have imagined it signaled the start of the worst-ever Ebola epidemic.

The outbreak that has swept through West Africa like wildfire, killing nearly 5,000 people so far and threatening to infect tens of thousands in the coming weeks, smoldered undetected for months before erupting onto the world stage. The virus first took hold in a triangle-shaped forested area where the porous borders of Guinea, Liberia and Sierra Leone meet.

"Ground zero" for the outbreak was an impoverished area where people are constantly crossing into neighboring countries -- "a dream situation for a highly contagious virus," the World Health Organization said Tuesday.

The UN agency has tracked the first case back to a two-year-old boy Emile Ouamouno who contracted an unknown illness in December in the remote Guinean village of Meliandou. Emile Ouamouno, who lived in the picturesque forest village with his parents and three sisters, including 4-year-old Philomene. The boy fell sick last December with a mysterious illness that caused fever, black stools and vomiting and died two days later. About a week after his death, Philomene got sick and died. She was shortly followed by the children's pregnant mother and grandmother.

It would be months before international health officials identified little Emile as West Africa's "patient zero" in a deadly outbreak that continues to double in size every few weeks. So far, Ebola has been blamed for the deaths of nearly 5,000 people among more than 10,000 cases, the vast majority in West Africa.

"Emile loved to dance and Philomene liked to carry little babies on her back and pretend she was a mom," said Suzanne Beukes of UNICEF, who spoke with their father Etienne during her trip earlier this month to Meliandou, a village without any health facility, more than a two-hour drive from the capital, Conakry.

Etienne burned the clothing and blankets of his two children killed by Ebola, but kept the small red radio that Emile often asked him to switch on so he could dance to the music.

The bodies of Emile, Philomene and their mother are buried next to the two-room house where Etienne lives with his second wife and three daughters.

"When we asked him what Emile was like, his face changed," Beukes said. "It's almost like a mask had been removed and the trauma of what he had been through became very visible."

Beukes said Ebola has killed at least 14 people in the settlement of about 500, though health officials say the actual case count is probably two to four times higher than official numbers.

The virus is believed to have been passed on by fruit bats, which are thought to be the natural reservoir of Ebola. Hunters are thought to have caught bat-infected monkeys, antelope, or squirrels for meat.

After it became clear that Guinea was dealing with an outbreak of Ebola, the WHO's top expert on the virus, Pierre Formenty, traced back the first 14 cases, all of whom were already dead.

"In an ominous hint of what would come, one of these first cases died in Sierra Leone," the UN agency said, referring to how easily the virus has managed to spread between countries.

Even as the bodies piled up, health officials were unable to identify the killer as Ebola, a virus never before seen in west Africa.

- 'No alarm bells rang' -

"Alarm bells might have gone off had any doctor or health official in the country ever seen a case of Ebola. No one had. No alarm bells rang," the WHO said.

Adding to the confusion, the affected area is notorious for outbreaks of cholera and other illnesses, and many Ebola symptoms are similar to endemic local diseases.

The virus continued its silent but lethal spread until staff from the Doctors Without Borders (MSF) charity sent a report on the strange deaths to a top expert in Geneva, who suspected a haemorrhagic fever, perhaps Ebola.

After spreading undetected for three months, the outbreak was finally officially declared on March 23.

Only four days later, the virus had made its way to Guinea's capital Conakry, as "new cases hit like sparks from a fire landing on dry grass," the WHO said.

"The brushfire had begun," the UN health agency said, describing the "heart-breaking" pattern that followed.

On three occasions, Guinea appeared set to quell the outbreak and began the count-down for the 21-day incubation period to pass without any new cases.

But each time, "vigilance eased and the sense of emergency lapsed," the agency said, explaining how Guinea -- which has now recorded more than 1,000 cases and 632 deaths -- and the international community let down their guard.

This allowed the virus, one of the deadliest known to man, to spread freely to neighboring Liberia and Sierra Leone.

Liberia was quickly engulfed by the outbreak and is today by far the hardest-hit country, with almost 1,600 deaths.

Things got off to a better start in Sierra Leone, which confirmed its first Ebola case on May 24 and put the patient in isolation in Kenema the next day.

She recovered without infecting anyone else at the hospital.

"All the right precautions were taken," WHO said.

But the person who infected her -- a widely-respected traditional healer in Sierra Leone who had treated Ebola patients from Guinea -- was not tracked down, and is believed to be linked to as many as 365 Ebola deaths.

By mid-June, an explosive outbreak was underway in Sierra Leone's third city of Kenema, and soon also in the capital Freetown. The country has now recorded almost 600 people killed by Ebola.

Five researchers who helped to trace the cases to the healer were felled by the virus before their study was published.

Many other health professionals have also died in the country, including one of the world's leading experts on haemorrhagic fevers, Sheik Humarr Kahn.

2 BUSTING THE MYTHS

As the Ebola virus continues to spread in Sierra Leone, Liberia and Guinea, health officials are concerned that myths and misinformation may continue to spread too.

The virus has claimed more than 4000 lives so far, and experts say a key part of fighting the disease is to make sure people are armed with the facts.

We take a look at some of the rumours surrounding Ebola - from false claims of miracle onions to condensed milk.

MYTH: Salt Water Or Raw Onions Can Protect You

Raw onions are not secret weapons against the disease.

Salt water simply cannot stop you from catching Ebola.

In fact drinking salty water, particularly in hot conditions, can be dangerous.

The WHO says at least two people in Nigeria died from this practice, believing it could prevent them from getting the disease.

And health workers in Guinea have been asked whether eating raw onions once a day for three days or a daily drink of condensed milk can keep Ebola away.

Though having a diet of nutritious food can keep you generally healthy, raw onions and milk do not stop you getting the infection.

Ebola is spread through close contact with the bodily fluids of someone who has the disease - for example the virus is present in vomit, urine, tears or saliva.

People can help protect themselves by avoiding close contact with anyone who has signs or symptoms of the disease.

MYTH: You Cannot Catch Ebola From A Deceased Person

Close contact with deceased persons should be avoided.

Even when someone has died of Ebola, the virus may still be present.

Health officials are concerned the disease might spread during traditional funeral practices that involve close contact with the deceased person.

The WHO says people who have died of Ebola must be handled using strong protective clothing and gloves, and they must be buried immediately.

Officials recommend burials should be conducted by people who have had training in how to stop the infection from spreading further.

MYTH: It Cannot Be Caught Through Sexual Contact

If a man has Ebola, the virus may be present in his bodily fluids - including his semen.

And Ebola can remain in semen for seven weeks after recovery - even if doctors have confirmed there is no longer any viral particles in the blood.

Anyone who has had Ebola should avoid sexual intercourse or use condoms during this time.

MYTH: Health Care Workers Brought The Disease Into Affected Countries

There has been some mistrust towards healthcare workers

There have been recent reports that health workers in Guinea were attacked because residents believed they had brought Ebola into the country.

But this was not true.

The WHO says the initial source of the Ebola virus was likely to be human contact with wild animals through hunting, butchering and preparing meat from infected wild animals.

It is possible, for example, that close contact with infected bats, shrews or small rodents passed on the disease.

During this outbreak, experts have advised people not to hunt or eat this type of bush meat.

MYTH: Expensive Hand Sanitizers Are Needed To Kill The Disease

Washing your hands can help stop the spread of Ebola.

Frequent hand washing with soap and water is recommended, particularly if you are in contact with an Ebola patient or his/her surroundings.

Alcohol gel can be useful but if the hands are visibly dirty it is important to wash your hands with clean water and soap, health officials say.

3 MAPPING THE OUTBREAK

The Ebola outbreak in West Africa was first reported in March 2014, and has rapidly become the deadliest occurrence of the disease since its discovery in 1976.

In fact, the current epidemic which has swept across the region has now killed more than all other known Ebola outbreaks combined.

Up to 28 September, 3,338 people had been reported as having died from the disease in four countries; Liberia, Guinea, Sierra Leone and Nigeria. The total number of reported cases is in excess of 7,178.

The World Health Organisation (WHO) admits the figures are underestimates, warning that there could be as many as 20,000 cases by November if efforts to tackle the outbreak are not stepped up.

Ebola deaths

Up to 25 October, 2014

4,922

Deaths (probable, confirmed and suspected)

2,705 Liberia

926 Guinea

1,281 Sierra Leone

8 Nigeria

1 Mali

1 USA

Source: WHO

The first case of the deadly virus diagnosed on US soil was announced on 1 October. The unnamed patient is thought to have contracted the virus in Liberia before travelling to the United States almost two weeks ago.

He had not displayed any symptoms of the disease until 24 September, five days after his arrival.

Emergency declared

In August, the United Nations health agency declared an "international public health emergency", saying that a co-ordinated response was essential to halt the spread of the virus.

However, WHO director general Margaret Chan said in September that the "number of patients is moving far faster than the capacity to manage them".

Despite attempts to deploy more health workers and open new Ebola treatment centres in the worst-affected countries, the WHO said that there was still a significant lack of beds in Sierra Leone and Liberia, with more than 2,000 needed.

Country	Existing bed capacity	Newly funded beds	Extra beds still required
Source: WHO, 24 September 2014			
Guinea	180	0	40
Liberia	315	440	1,550
Sierra Leone	323	297	532

The outbreaks in Senegal and Nigeria have been "pretty much contained", as there have been no new cases reported there since 5 September.

According to the WHO, the situation in Guinea also appeared to be stabilising however there appears no indication of a reversal in Sierra Leone and Liberia.

Transmission is continuing in urban areas, with the surge in Liberia driven mainly by a sharp increase in the number of cases reported in the capital, Monrovia.

The situation in Sierra Leone also continues to deteriorate with a sharp increase in the number of newly-reported cases in the capital, Freetown, and its neighbouring districts of Port Loko, Bombali, and Moyamba, which are were placed under quarantine on 25 September.

That means that five of Sierra Leone's 15 districts are on lockdown, with more than a third of the population of six million no longer able to move freely.

Current outbreak

Figures accurate from 26-29 September, depending on country. Death toll in Liberia includes probable, suspect and confirmed cases, while in Sierra Leone and Guinea only confirmed cases are shown

Researchers from the New England Journal of Medicine have traced the outbreak to a two-year-old girl, who died on 6 December 2013 in Meliandou, a small village in south-eastern Guinea.

In March, hospital staff alerted Guinea's Ministry of Health and then the charity Medecins Sans Frontieres (MSF). They reported a mysterious disease in the south-eastern regions of Gueckedou, Macenta, Nzerekore, and Kissidougou.

It caused fever, diarrhoea and vomiting. It also had a high death rate. Of the first 86 cases, 59 people died.

The WHO later confirmed the disease as Ebola.

Disease spreads

Gueckedou is a major regional trading centre and, by the end of March, Ebola had crossed the border into Liberia and it was confirmed in Sierra Leone in May.

In June, MSF described the Ebola outbreak as out of control.

Nigeria had its first case of the disease in July and in the same month two leading doctors died from Ebola in Liberia and Sierra Leone. Senegal reported its first case of Ebola on 29 August. A young man from Guinea had travelled to Senegal despite having been infected with the virus, officials said.

The WHO has published updates on the spread of the virus in each of the countries affected.

The figures given are for "confirmed, probable and suspected" cases and deaths. They have occasionally been revised down to take account of changes in the countries' reporting methods, for example by excluding the "suspected" cases.

2014 outbreak in context

Ebola occurs in regions of sub-Saharan Africa, though normally fewer than 500 cases occur each year.

No cases at all were reported between 1979 and 1994, however, the 2014 outbreak dwarfs all previous outbreaks.

How Ebola Came To Nigeria

Ebola victim, Patrick Sawyer, 40, who died of the deadly virus in Lagos, Nigeria, on July 25 was scheduled to return to the United States in August.

His wife, Decontee Sawyer, said her husband was to return for two of their daughters' birthdays.

Decontee and the children lived in Coon Rapids, Michigan.

Patrick Sawyer died on Friday July 25, 2014 after suffering extreme bouts of vomiting and diarrhea on a flight from Liberia to Nigeria

Decontee said her husband had planned to return to their Coon Rapids home in August to attend two of his three daughters' birthdays, Minnesota's KSTP-TV reported.

The grieving widow said she hoped her husband's death served as a wake-up call about the global threat of the virus, which had already killed any people globally.

"It's a global problem because Patrick could've easily come home with Ebola It's close; it's at our front door. It knocked down my front door," Decontee said.

Sawyer lived in Minnesota for about a decade before returning to Liberia in 2008 to work as a finance minister, KSTP-TV reported.

His wife said he was beloved in their local Liberian community.

Nigerian Diplomat, Olu-Ibukun Koye Who Took Ebola To Port Harcourt

He was one of the first who made contact with the late Liberian, Patrick Sawyer.

Recall that Olu defied instructions and ran to Port Harcourt to meet late doctor Iyke Enemuo who treated him in a hotel.

Shortly after he was treated, he returned to Lagos where he was certified Ebola free.

Ironically, Dr Iyke fell ill and died. His wife opened up and his corpse which was taken to a mortuary was tested positive for Ebola.

The late doctor's wife who is infected too is currently quarantined in Lagos.

She has a 3 month old baby.

According to reports, Olu may face manslaughter charges.

How Did Ebola Get Into USA

A Liberian man is the first person to be diagnosed with the deadly Ebola virus on US soil. So how did he arrive undetected and what are the risks to Americans?

The outbreak gripping the World now is the World's worst, killing 4,922 people so far.

There have been 10,000 confirmed cases, with Liberia, Sierra Leone and Guinea suffering the most.

This case in the US is thought to be the first outside West Africa involving this strain of Ebola.

Who is the new patient in the US?

The person diagnosed with the virus while in the US.

Thomas Eric Duncan, a Liberian national, tested positive in Dallas, Texas, on 30 September.

He arrived in the US to visit relatives on 20 September and is now in a serious condition in an isolation unit at a hospital in Dallas.

Is he the first person in the US to have Ebola? No, a small number of American aid workers who contracted the virus while abroad have recovered after flying back to the US for treatment. But Mr Duncan is the first diagnosed within the US.

Three of the aid workers were colleagues at the same hospital in Liberia. Kent Brantly and Nancy Writebol were flown back to Atlanta for treatment, while Rick Sacra, a family doctor from Massachusetts, recovered in Nebraska.

Ms Writebol said resources at the hospital where they worked were insufficient to protect workers.

A month after returning to the US, Ms Writebol was well enough to speak to reporters.

Do we know how Mr Duncan was infected? It is believed he came into contact with an Ebola infectious woman in Liberia on 15 September, according to a report by the New York Times.

Mr Duncan is said to have helped take her to hospital, but she was later turned away due to lack of space in the Ebola treatment ward. He helped to carry her home, where she died hours later.

Williams' brother, Sonny Boy, also later displayed symptoms of Ebola and died en route to a local hospital.

How did an infected person come into the US undetected? Mr Duncan was screened for Ebola symptoms at Roberts International Airport, located near the Liberian capital of Monrovia.

He displayed no signs of the virus and was allowed to board an SN Brussels Airlines flight to Brussels, Belgium.

From there, he flew to Washington Dulles and then on to Dallas-Fort Worth, arriving on 20 September.

Binyah Kesselly, chairman of the board of the Liberia Airport Authority, said they had screened 10,000 passengers since July, but it would be "nearly impossible" to identify a person as infected with the Ebola virus if they were not showing symptoms.

Are the passengers on his flight in danger? The Centers for Disease Control and Prevention (CDC) do not plan to monitor passengers on Mr Duncan's flights.

According to CDC Director Thomas Frieden, Mr Duncan was not considered infectious at that time and posed "zero risk of transmission" to those on the aircraft.

Should he have been diagnosed earlier?

Mr Duncan sought medical attention at Texas Health Presbyterian Hospital on 25 September, where hospital officials said he displayed a low grade fever and abdominal pain. Basic blood tests were performed, but he was not screened for the Ebola virus.

A nurse asked Mr Duncan if he had travelled from Africa, and he said he had, but that detail was not fully communicated to the medical staff, an oversight the hospital now says it "regrets".

Mr Duncan was given antibiotics and a pain reliever and sent home, where his condition worsened, says his sister.

On 28 September, a friend of Mr Duncan's contacted the CDC for advice, and was instructed to call the Texas Department of Health, who sent an ambulance.

Are people he has been in contact with at risk?

There was a four-day period between Mr Duncan developing symptoms and being put in isolation in hospital.

So officials are identifying and monitoring all the people he came into contact with. If they show no symptoms after 21 days, they are considered to be uninfected.

Up to 20 people, including five children, are being monitored after coming into contact with him, mostly at the house where he stayed.

According to a statement from the local school district in Dallas, Mr Duncan came into contact with five children from four different schools.

Mr Frieden said it is possible a family member who came in direct contact with the patient may develop Ebola in the coming weeks.

4 FIVE WAYS TO BREAK THE EPIDEMIC

With the worst-ever outbreak of Ebola revealing woefully inadequate health systems in West Africa, especially in those countries recovering from civil war, the international response and leadership of the World Health Organization (WHO) has also come in for criticism.

Announcing US plans, President Barack Obama said the outbreak was "a threat to global security" which required a "global response".

So, what would bring the epidemic under control? Here are five things officials say would help:

1) More Treatment Centres

All agree this is key as the real number of cases is believed to be much higher than the 4,366 recorded.

Victims in Liberia - the country worst-affected by Ebola - are spreading the virus, some dying on the streets, because there is not enough room at isolation clinics set up to treat infected patients.

President Obama's plan to send 3,000 troops to build 17 healthcare facilities and train health workers has been met with some relief, especially in Liberia where most of this deployment will go.

But it may take weeks before the first US beds are operational, and the WHO has confirmed that there are no free beds anywhere in Liberia at present.

People with Ebola symptoms in Liberia cannot get beds in centres dealing with the virus

The aid group Medecins Sans Frontieres (MSF) has urged other countries to "deploy their civil defence and military assets, and medical teams, to contain the epidemic".

Last week, the UK announced it would set up a 65-bed treatment centre for infected medical staff in Sierra Leone, and France has put a team of about 20 experts on rotation to Guinea.

But Philippe Maughan, who works for Echo, the humanitarian aid branch of the European Commission, thinks MSF's expectations may be too high.

"If it thinks there is a sort of foreign legion ready to deploy for this outbreak, there isn't," Dr Maughan says.

"Ebola is a very specific virus for which even specialists in infectious diseases are not necessarily skilled."

2) Home Care

Until promised treatment centres are set up, this will be the best attempt to stem infections - especially in Liberia.

Under broad medical supervision, affected communities would learn how to provide basic care using rehydration and painkillers.

"It won't be possible without the participation of the community," warns Tarik Jasarevic, a WHO spokesman.

Gaining the trust of fearful communities is key

This will include breaking down the fear of people wearing protective suits. But it is a risky move.

"The need in personnel to have this work is big; supervision and discipline are key," says Dr Maughan.

"Some will fail and some will work. It's not ideal, this is a last resort."

MSF warns it will only work in the early stages of treatment.

"As soon as their family member shows more severe symptoms, like bleeding, they will seek to bring them in a treatment centre anyway," says Brice de la Vigne, MSF's director of operations.

3) Air Bridge And Medevac System

Guinea, Sierra Leone and Liberia, the worst-hit states, have been isolated because of flight bans and borders being shut - despite WHO recommendations to the contrary.

It has dealt a blow to their economies and food security will soon become an issue.

Aid agencies are lobbying states to grant them humanitarian corridors.

President Obama has promised to develop an air bridge to get supplies into affected countries faster.

Senegal, where many UN agencies and non-governmental organisations (NGOs) have their regional offices, is expected to become a logistical hub.

The authorities there have officially agreed to it but, sources say, remain reluctantly slow in turning the theory into practice.

"I understand the concerns from the Senegalese government; Ebola was brought to Nigeria by an airline passenger after all, but we need to get equipment in these countries and we need to get staff in and out," Dr Maughan says.

The evacuation of infected medical staff is also an issue, potentially limiting volunteers.

4) Preparation Elsewhere

Don't wait until there is a confirmed case to get ready and make sure what looks good on paper can work on the ground, is the warning to countries in the region.

When it arrived in Nigeria, people were spooked, one diplomat told the BBC.

"If the CDC (Centre for Disease Control and Prevention) hadn't sent 50 experts to Nigeria, they would not have it under control," Dr Maughan says.

Medical kits are now being dispatched throughout the region and some countries have started public awareness campaigns.

Medical agencies believe that if there are more cases in Senegal, where 67 people are still under surveillance after coming into contact with an infected Guinean student, the outbreak could be quickly stopped.

But concerns remain over the capacity to act quickly in countries most at risk - Mali, Guinea-Bissau and Ivory Coast.

"We are working with the authorities in Mali to get all the 86 health centres and hospitals we sponsor there ready," says Alexis Smigielski, head of the Dakar-based medical charity Alima.

5) Vaccines

At least two experimental vaccines are looking promising and could be made available in West Africa in November if trials are conclusive.

Injections would be given to medical staff as a priority.

"It holds quite a lot of hope," says Dr Maughan.

5 FIVE WAYS TO AVOID THE DEADLY VIRUS

Ebola is one of the world's most deadly viruses but is not airborne, so cannot be caught like flu. Medical experts say avoiding it should be quite easy if you follow these tips:

1. Soap and Water

Wash your hands often with soap and clean water - and use clean towels to dry them. This can be difficult in slum and rural areas where there is not always direct access to clean water - but it is an effective way to kill the virus. Ordinary soap is all that's needed.

Shaking hands should also generally be avoided, Dr Unni Krishnan of Plan International told BBC Africa, because Ebola spreads quickly when people come into contact with an infected person's body fluids and symptoms can take a while to show. Other forms of greeting are being encouraged, he says.

2. No Touching

So if you suspect someone of having Ebola, do not touch them. This may seem cruel when you see a loved one in pain and you want to hug and nurse them, but body fluids - urine and stools, vomit, blood, nasal mucus, saliva, tears, sperm and vaginal secretion - can all pass on the virus.

An infected person's symptoms include fever, muscle and joint pain, sore throat, headache and fatigue - followed by nausea, vomiting and diarrhoea, which may include blood.

Encourage them to seek help from a medical professional or health centre as soon as possible. It is also advisable not to touch the clothes or bedclothes of Ebola patients - and Medecins Sans Frontieres advises that such sheets and even mattresses be burnt.

3. Avoid Dead Bodies

If you think someone has died from Ebola, do not touch their body, even as part of a burial ceremony. When someone has died, you can still catch Ebola from their body as it ejects fluids that make it even more contagious than that of a sick person.

Organise for a specialised team to deal with the body as quickly as possible as it is risky to leave a dead body for any length of time in a cramped living area.

4. No Bushmeat

Avoid hunting, touching and eating bushmeat such as bats, monkeys and chimpanzees, as scientists believe this is how the virus was first transmitted to humans.

Even if a certain wild animal is a delicacy in your region, avoid it as its meat or blood may be contaminated. Make sure all food is cooked properly.

5. Don't Panic

Spreading rumours increases fear. Do not be scared of health workers - they are there to help and a clinic is the best place for a person to recover - they will be rehydrated and receive pain relief.

About half of the people infected in the current outbreak have died. There have been cases of medics being attacked and people being abandoned when they are suspected of having Ebola - even when they are suffering from something else.

"Prevention is the best way to deal with Ebola, so stop rumours and do not panic; it is possible to reduce the suffering and save lives," Dr Krishnan says.

How Not To Catch Ebola

- Avoid direct contact with sick patients as the virus is spread through contaminated body fluids
- Wear goggles to protect eyes.
- Clothing and clinical waste should be incinerated and any medical equipment that needs to be kept should be decontaminated.
- People who recover from Ebola should abstain from sex or use condoms for three months.

Ebola Virus Disease (EVD):

- Symptoms include high fever, bleeding and central nervous system damage
- Fatality rate can reach 90% - but current outbreak has mortality rate of about 55%
- Incubation period is two to 21 days
- There is no proven vaccine or cure
- Supportive care such as rehydrating patients who have diarrhoea and vomiting can help recovery
- Fruit bats, a delicacy for some West Africans, are considered to be virus's natural host

With supportive care, patients can survive - like this man in Sierra Leone - and their blood may help treat others

However, it could take several months to reach a production that would respond to the scale of demand.

The WHO has also indicated that people who have survived can now provide blood to treat patients who are sick.

But the UN health agency has warned that current lab experiments should not distract from the actual needs on the ground.

6 HOW BAD CAN IT GET?

One Horrifying Sentence Explains Why Ebola Has Spread So Quickly

A vivid and terrifying story in The New York Times helps explain why the Ebola virus has spread so quickly across West Africa.

The hospitals in the region simply aren't equipped to deal with the disease at the rate that it's spreading. They don't have the right tools or resources to care for existing patients, let alone stem the spread of the disease.

One sentence from the Times story illustrates this well. Adam Nossiter writes from Sierra Leone that at one hospital isolation ward in Makeni, **"Nurses, some not wearing gloves and others in street clothes, clustered by the door as pools of the patients' bodily fluids spread to the threshold."**

Ebola is spread via bodily fluids, putting healthcare workers who are not properly protected at extraordinary risk.

From the Times story:

A worker kicked another man on the floor to see if he was still alive. The man's foot moved and the team kept going. It was 1:30 in the afternoon.

In the next ward, a 4-year-old girl lay on the floor in urine, motionless, bleeding from her mouth, her eyes open. A corpse lay in the corner — a young woman, legs akimbo, who had died overnight.

A small child stood in a cot watching as the team took the body away, stepping around a little boy lying immobile next to black buckets of vomit. They sprayed the body, and the little girl on the floor, with chlorine as they left.

The nurses at these hospitals are "lightly trained and minimally protected" and Ebola patients are dying "surrounded by pools of infectious waste," Nossiter reports.

Daniel Bausch, a doctor and associate professor in the department of tropical medicine at Tulane, went to Sierra Leone in July and saw many of the same conditions.

He told Business Insider in August that in some hospitals, there is no running water, soap, or clean needles, which are all crucial to controlling the outbreak and preventing further spread of disease.

"The scale of this outbreak has just outstripped the resources," Bausch said.

Ebola begins with flu-like symptoms and in many cases escalates to internal and external bleeding and organ failure. The disease has a high fatality rate, especially in countries that are ill-equipped to care for infected patients.

The Centers for Disease Control and Prevention announced this week that the first case of Ebola had been diagnosed in the US, but we're much more well-positioned to prevent the spread of the disease.

The US has the resources to properly contain the virus, which spreads through bodily fluids, not the air.

West Africa is a different story. Ebola has killed 4,922 and infected at least 10,000 people in the region so far, and those numbers continue to climb.

"There are few signs yet that the [Ebola] epidemic in West Africa is being brought under control," the World Health Organization noted in its latest report.

It is also unclear when this outbreak will be over.

Officially the World Health Organization is saying the outbreak can be contained in six to nine months. But that is based on getting the resources to tackle the outbreak, which are currently stretched too thinly to contain Ebola as it stands.

There have been nearly 10,000 cases so far, cases are increasing exponentially and there is a potentially vulnerable population in Sierra Leone, Liberia and Guinea in excess of 20 million.

Ebola Death Rates 70% – WHO Study

New figures suggest 70% of those infected with Ebola in West Africa have died, higher than previously reported, says the World Health Organization.

Ebola infections will treble to 20,000 by November if efforts to tackle the outbreak are not stepped up, the UN agency has warned.

In the worst case scenario, cases in two nations could reach 1.4 million in January, according to a US estimate.

Experts said the US numbers were "somewhat pessimistic."

The world's largest outbreak of Ebola has caused 4,922 deaths so far, mainly in Guinea, Liberia, Nigeria, USA and Sierra Leone.

Outbreaks in Senegal and Nigeria were "pretty much contained", said the WHO.

Scientists have warned that swift action is needed to curb the exponential climb in the Ebola outbreak.

Two new estimates suggest that cases of Ebola could soar dramatically in the three countries with the majority of cases.

Projections published in The New England Journal of Medicine predict that by early November there will have been nearly 20,000 cases.

The analysis of confirmed cases also suggests death rates are higher than previously reported at about 70% of all cases, rather than 50%.

Dr Christopher Dye, Director of Strategy for WHO, said unless control measures improved quickly "these three countries will soon be reporting thousands of cases and deaths each week, projections that are similar to those of the Centers for Disease Control and Prevention (CDC)".

The CDC said that there could be up to 21,000 reported and unreported cases in Liberia and Sierra Leone alone by the end of this month.

In predictions released on Tuesday, the US health agency said cases could reach as many as 1.4 million by mid-January, if efforts to control the outbreak are not scaled up.

But experts cautioned that the numbers seemed "somewhat pessimistic" and did not account for infection control efforts already underway.

There Are No More Samples Of The Experimental Ebola Drug ZMapp

MADRID (AP) — Doctors treating a Spanish priest who was repatriated from West Africa on Monday after being diagnosed with the Ebola virus said there were no samples of experimental drug ZMapp available in the world right now, and they were considering alternative treatments.

The priest, Manuel Garcia Viejo, 69, was in serious condition and was suffering from dehydration, with kidney and liver complications, said Javier Rodriguez, chief health officer for the Madrid region.

Garcia Viejo, a medical director of the San Juan de Dios Hospital in Lunsar, Sierra Leone, was transferred to Madrid Carlos III hospital after being flown back from Sierra Leone in a medically-equipped military plane.

Mapp Biopharmaceutical, the company that makes ZMapp, says the drug's supplies are exhausted and that it takes months to make even a small batch.

With ZMapp unavailable, the hospital was looking into alternative medicines or the possibility of using blood serum from a cured patient, said Dr. Jose Ramon Arribas, of the Carlos III hospital.

Garcia Viejo is the second Spanish missionary to catch Ebola. Another priest, Miguel Pajares, 75, was flown back to Spain from Liberia on Aug. 7. Pajares began treatment with ZMapp, but died Aug. 12.

Ebola is blamed for the deaths of more than 4000 people in West Africa.

The Health Ministry said Garcia Viejo asked to be transferred back to Spain after testing positive for the deadly virus.

Failure Of Laws

The MSF boss further advised authorities in countries where the virus was endemic to reverse laws criminalising failure to report suspected cases, saying such measures had only heightened fear and unrest.

"Coercive measures, such as law criminalising the failure to report suspected cases and forced quarantines are driving people underground. This is leading to the concealment of cases, and is pushing the sick away from health systems,'' she said.

Despite the grim report, foreign volunteers are arriving worst- hit countries in trickles. Working with Ebola patients in Liberia, American paediatrician, Alan Jamison, treated as many people as he could as the country slipped into chaos. Each day, more patients showed up at the hospital's doors.

The deadly virus wasn't the only danger: Ebola was causing such fear that some Liberians were threatening to burn down the isolation unit with doctors and patients inside.

Jamison's medical missionary group pulled him out early as a precaution. Still, the 69-year-old retiree said he would return.

"This is where the need is," Jamison explained. "This is my calling.

Jamison isn't alone. Even after three American aid workers fell sick, many other doctors, nurses and other health care volunteers are on their way to West Africa, helping to staff hospitals and clinics and screen travellers to slow the epidemic's spread.

Why are so many willing to put themselves in harm's way?

"It's a call, a zeal, a devotion. It's an acceptance of a professional life outside the ordinary, with an element of adventure," said William Schaffner, an infectious disease specialist at the Vanderbilt University in Nashville, Tennessee.

Hospital volunteer, Nancy Writebol and Dr. Kent Brantly, were already in Liberia when the outbreak began, and decided to stay at the charity-run ELWA hospital in Monrovia to help. Richard Sacra, a 15-year ELWA veteran, immediately volunteered to leave his family in suburban Boston and return to the hospital when Writebol and Brantly got sick. Jamison also worked there.

All are committed to their cause. Like Jamison, Nancy Writebol and her husband, David, said that they would consider going back. Brantly said he could not return just yet, but would keep campaigning to end Ebola. Sacra also had no regrets, his wife said as the doctor was evacuated to the isolation unit in a Nebraska hospital.

"Once you go and you see the Lord at work, I mean, there's nothing else that you want to do," Nancy Writebol said.

These volunteers are passionate, but there's also a cold logic to their commitment: This epidemic that has killed 4,922 people and sickened 10,000 in five West African nations and USA won't end unless more experienced health care workers confront it directly.

Spread Of Virus

Ebola is being spread by people, in hospitals, homes and funerals. People catch the virus when they have direct contact with the blood or bodily fluids of those who are sick and dying, or already dead. At ELWA, Jamison trained workers how to protect themselves and the wider population.

The hospital in Monrovia is operated by Charlotte-based SIM USA, and includes more than 200 beds as well as the 50-bed isolation unit for Ebola patients.

Keeping those populations separate is essential, Jamison said, but is no simple matter. He trained workers to wear a mask and gloves and screen new patients from several feet away before they were allowed to enter. When patients showed signs of Ebola, a worker wearing a protective suit would be summoned to bring them to a holding area for evaluation and then to the isolation unit if necessary. But the screeners have to ask the right questions to bring out the truth in such a fearful environment, Jamison said.

And if anyone masking Ebola symptoms is allowed inside, they could expose many more people who don't routinely wear full-body protective suits.

"Sometimes I felt safer in the Ebola unit than in the hospital," Jamison said.

Most international aid organisations are quite familiar with the risks of sending health care workers into terrain plagued by war, political turmoil and disease. But this Ebola epidemic has posed serious and unique challenges.

"We're balancing tremendous need in a risky environment," said Joe DiCarlo, a vice-president at Jamison's sponsor, the Portland, Oregon-based Medical Teams International. It's a non-denominational Christian group that has been working in Liberia for 10 years, with 15 permanent medical staff in the country, including three Americans, supporting 240 clinics around the country.

"We are finding volunteers who want to go, even though they are fully aware of the situation," DiCarlo said. "We're getting the people we need, but I can't say we're overwhelmed with requests."

Liberia has the largest caseload and death toll, but many of its hospitals have been closed. There are just two large hospitals still operating in the country of four million people, said George Salloum, SIM's financial officer.

About 250 people work at ELWA – most of them Liberian. They usually have between three and seven American doctors who serve two to three years.

Right now, there's only one American doctor left on-site.

After some airlines stopped flying to countries affected by the outbreak, it's been much harder to get enough medical supplies to keep up with demand, including critical protective gear to keep its doctors and nurses safe. ELWA is no exception. Staffers go through thousands of disposable protective suits a week. Salloum said they recently received a shipment of protective gear, but they're running short of other supplies, including the intravenous fluids and electrolytes needed to keep Ebola victims alive long enough for their bodies' immune systems to fight the virus.

"We just take for granted how easy it is in America to get these things," he said.

The number of patients in the Ebola isolation unit fluctuates – but is usually close to capacity, he said.

No Going Back

With so much need, SIM has no plans to pull out, said Will Elphick, the group's director for Liberia.

"You have to weigh out the risk compared with what you feel you can do with a situation where there is so much need," Elphick said. "We still want to support our Liberian colleagues."

That will require more supplies, and volunteers.

More Women Than Men Are Dying From Ebola

The current Ebola outbreak may ultimately infect as many as 20,000 people and a disproportionate number of those cases will be women, experts say.

Since this strain of the disease first hit Guinea in May, 4500 people have succumbed to Ebola, which has been rapidly making its way through four countries in West Africa and US. More women than men are contracting the disease though, since they traditionally serve as health care workers and are the ones who are expected to look after ill family members, according to UNICEF.

Women account for 55 to 60 percent of victims who have died from Ebola in the current epidemic in Liberia, Guinea and Sierra Leone, according UNICEF.

But figures may actually be even higher.

Health teams in Liberia recently reported that women made up 75 percent of victims who were infected or died from Ebola, The Washington Post reported.

The outbreak is being attributed to the consumption of infected bush meat -- the meat of wild animals -- which many rely on for their livelihood and as their main source of protein, according to Irin News.

The disease spreads when there is direct contact with the blood, body fluids and tissues of infected animals or people, which is more of a risk for women who are expected to spearhead taking care of ill family members and preparing for funerals, according to UNICEF.

"Women are the caregivers – if a kid is sick, they say, 'Go to your mom," Sia Nyama Koroma, first lady of Sierra Leone, told The Washington Post. "Most of the time when there is a death in the family, it's the woman who prepares the funeral, usually an aunt or older female relative."

A key reason this outbreak, and ones similar to it, continue to hit West Africa is because -- across the board -- both men and women are reluctant to seek medical care. They've developed strained relationships with healthcare workers and century-old traditions mandate that the ill be taken of at home, Raphael Frankfurter, executive director of Wellbody Alliance -- a group that provides free healthcare in Sierra Leone -- told HuffPost earlier this month.

This burden of tending to the sick, however, is the one that women have to bare.

"If a man is sick, the woman can easily bathe him but the man cannot do so," Marpue Spear, executive director of the Women's NGO Secretariat of Liberia, told Foreign Policy. "Traditionally, women will take care of the men as compared to them taking care of the women."

Helping to change these perspectives is what will finally put an end to these devastating outbreaks, Frankfurter said.

Currently, because there is so much confrontation associated with the disease -- the military will surround an infected person's home and healthcare workers often don't respect a patient's ancient traditions -- Ebola victims don't want to seek out help from clinics.

But if these relationships could be mended and West African men and women would be more open to getting treated at clinics, then these epidemics could be stopped before they spread to this insidious level, Frankfurter believes.

The 23-year-old aid worker saw firsthand how this methodology actually works.

After a woman in Kona, Sierra Leone, tended to a funeral, she became infected and died from the disease.

Wellbody Alliance then went out into the community to find the 35 people she had been in contact with and did so in a compassionate way, Frankfurter said.

7 WHY EBOLA IS SO DANGEROUS

Low Survival Rates

The chance of survival is almost zero, especially in Africa. It kills 90 per cent of those infected with the virus. Death is certain if the patient starts bleeding. Bleeding, of course, is its "trademark".

From a medical point, any one that contracts this disease should be isolated –to wait for death! It is sad! It kills faster than AIDS, and in an equally dramatic way. Because of its mode of transmission, you cannot bury dead patients in the usual way — patients, dead or alive, are absolutely avoided! Dead bodies are equally infectious.

It is almost incurable.

The problem is that there is no drug yet for treatment or vaccine for prevention. Four different viruses cause this disease. At least, we have some drugs for HIV/AIDS patients, to help them live longer and better. The treatment offered for Ebola Virus Disease is for the person to die better and more peacefully. The vaccines we have can only prevent monkeys and mice from the disease! Antiviral do not work.

It Is Highly Contagious

HIV/AIDS requires blood transmission or intimate contact for transmission; this disease requires contact with body. Transmission is by coming in contact with body fluids from diarrhoea, vomiting, and bleeding. Doctors and medical staff attending to the patients wear protective kits from head to toe, making them look like astronauts heading for the moon! HIV is highest among commercial sex workers and gays; the people with the highest risk of Ebola Viral Disease are medical workers, their families, and their friends. Hunters that encounter monkeys and bats, and marketers of bush-meats should be careful.

No Definite Way To Protect Yourself

There is ABC of HIV/AIDS prevention. There are ways of preventing malaria. But preventing Ebola Virus Disease is not specific or clear-cut. You are advised to wash your hands frequently with soap and water, avoid contact with infected people (and their secretions and blood), and avoid contact with objects contaminated by infected people. Prevention is by hygiene!

Why Ebola Differs From Other Viruses

The Ebola Virus Disease is the enemy knocking at the door of many West African countries and the entire world and its effects are fast spreading.

Unlike other viruses, such as the Hepatitis A, B,C, which can stay in the body fluids of an infected person for 15 years without any symptoms, the Ebola virus, which symptoms include bleeding from the mouth and anus, can kill its victims within days .

A professor of Epidemiology and Community Health Science, University of Ilorin, Kwara State, Nigeria, Tanimola Akande, describes the Ebola virus, which is ravaging Guinea, Sierra Leone and Liberia and has killed a nurse in Nigeria, as the biggest health challenge facing the sub region at present.

Akande says that its mode of transmission is a major reason why it is deadlier than most viruses.

He says, "That Ebola has no cure is not the reason why it is deadly.HIV also has no cure, yet it does not kill all its victims, if it is properly managed. Ebola is deadlier because it is easy to contract; it is in all the body fluids of an infected individual as its infection can be through saliva, blood, sweat, sperm, excreta, body tissue. It can also be contracted by touching the surface an infected person has touched."

"Also, the natural host for Ebola is fruit bats, chimpanzees and other forest animals that many eat daily in different parts of the country. You can get it just by coming in contact with the blood of an infected animal. Any virus that can be contracted through food has the potential to wipe off many lives."

The physician, who says that Ebola virus has very tricky symptoms, which often mimic that of common illness, such as malaria, dengue, lassa and typhoid fever, notes that many health workers may have already come in contact with an infected patient without knowing it.

He adds, "When a patient comes to your hospital and presents you with symptoms, such as fever, headache, general body pain, you are likely not to wear gloves or biohazards suits before treating the patient. That is the tricky part. You are infected before you know it is Ebola."

To contain the transmission of the disease, Akande urges Nigerians to stop eating bush meat, as well as to wash their hands and fruits regularly before eating.

He also advises health workers to wear protective kits always while attending to their patients.

Akande states, "We have been talking about HIV/AIDS, but Ebola is deadlier than HIV/AIDS. People who have HIV live for years if they take their drugs but any contact with an infected Ebola person is almost a death sentence because the virus has no vaccines, and no drugs. The best one can get is only palliative management".

Ebola is the nightmare virus. It is feared as the second coming of the plagues of the 1400s. Why is this one virus so much more deadly than other viruses? Simply put, experts list five reasons why everyone must watch out for this virus.

World Losing The Battle —MSF

The International President, Medecins Sans Frontieres, Dr. Joanne Liu, has warned that the world may be losing the battle to stop the spread of the Ebola Virus Disease.

An international non-governmental organisation, the MSF, has provided medical aid in countries facing conflicts and developing countries since 1971 when it was founded by some French medical doctors and journalists in the wake of the Biafran secession.

Speaking to United Nations member states on Friday, Liu however declared that the provision of mobile laboratories and dedicated air bridges as well as building a regional network of field hospitals to treat suspected or infected medical personnel could still save the day.

According to her, developments in the aftermath of the outbreak of the EVD in West Africa are overwhelming just as she posited that the disease posed a transnational threat.

Liu said, "Six months into the worst Ebola epidemic in history, the world is losing the battle to contain it. Leaders are failing to come to grips with this transnational threat. In West Africa, cases and deaths continue to surge. Riots are breaking out. Isolation centres are overwhelmed. Health workers on the front lines are becoming infected and are dying in shocking numbers.

"Others have fled in fear, leaving people without care for even the most common illnesses. Entire systems have crumbled. Ebola treatment centres are reduced to places where people go to die alone, where little more than palliative care is offered.

"It is impossible to keep up with the sheer number of infected people pouring into facilities. In Sierra Leone, infectious bodies are rotting in the streets."

She also decried the slow response and attention given by governments and foreign aid donors around the world to the outbreak.

"I stand here today, as the president of a medical humanitarian organisation on the front lines of this outbreak since it emerged. My colleagues have cared for more than two thirds of the officially declared infected patients. Even as we have doubled our staff over the last month, I can tell you that they are completely overwhelmed.

"Medecins Sans Frontieres has been ringing alarm bells for months, but the response has been too little, too late. The outbreak began six months ago, but was only declared a 'Public Health Emergency of International Concern' on August 8. While funding announcements, roadmaps, and finding vaccines and treatments are welcome, they will not stop the epidemic today. We have been losing for the past six months. We must win over the next three. And we can,'' she said.

Ebola Mutation 'Presents Nightmare Scenario'

Virologists may not be publicly talking about the possibility that the Ebola virus could someday mutate into an airborne strain, writes Michael T Osterholm in the New York Times, but it's something they are "definitely considering in private".

The director of the Center for Infectious Disease Research and Policy at the University of Minnesota says that the virus - which currently can only be transmitted through contact with bodily fluids - has proven to be "notoriously sloppy in replicating", which increases the chances that it could turn into something more contagious.

"Why are public officials afraid to discuss this?" he asks. "They don't want to be accused of screaming 'fire!' in a crowded theatre - as I'm sure some will accuse me of doing. But the risk is real, and until we consider it, the world will not be prepared to do what is necessary to end the epidemic."

The second disturbing scenario he envisions is if the Ebola virus is brought to a more densely populated area of the world, where it would be more difficult to contain.

According to the World Health Organisation, the virus has already killed around 4,922 people. It is now predicting that more than 20,000 may contract the virus before the current outbreak is over.

"What happens when an infected person yet to become ill travels by plane to Lagos, Nairobi, Kinshasa or Mogadishu - or even Karachi, Jakarta, Mexico City or Dhaka?" he asks. The more people who get infected, he says, the greater the opportunities for mutation.

"The current Ebola virus' hyper-evolution is unprecedented; there has been more human-to-human transmission in the past four months than most likely occurred in the last 500 to 1,000 years," he writes.

To prevent this, Osterholm says, the United Nations should be put in charge of overseeing containment of the outbreak by managing air supply chains, providing hospital beds and training medical staff.

Waiting for a vaccine isn't a realistic solution, he concludes. By the time one is developed, the disease could be in "our own backyards".

Although Osterholm paints a dark picture - and it's not the first time he's taken to a major daily newspaper to do so - other public health professionals are unconvinced. Scott Gottlieb, former deputy director of the US Food and Drug Administration, writes in Forbes that it is very unlikely that the Ebola virus would ever mutate into an airborne version.

"It would be unusual for a virus to transform in a way that changes its mode of infection," he writes. "Of the 23 known viruses that cause serious disease in man, none are known to have mutated in ways that changed how they infect humans."

Tara C Smith, writing for ScienceBlogs, says that diseases similar to Ebola have already appeared in the US and have been easily controlled. She adds that she is much more concerned with "ordinary" viruses like influenza and measles.

"Ebola is exotic and its symptoms can be terrifying, but also much easier to contain by people who know their stuff," she concludes.

8 ECONOMIC AND SOCIAL IMPACT

With more than 4,000 reported deaths from Ebola in West Africa and the world, the virus continues to be an urgent health crisis, but it is also having a devastating impact on the economies of Guinea, Liberia and Sierra Leone.

"The economy has been deflated by 30% because of Ebola," Sierra Leone's Agriculture Minister Joseph Sam Sesay told the BBC.

He said President Ernest Bai Koroma revealed this staggering and depressing news to ministers at a special cabinet meeting. "The agricultural sector is the most impacted in terms of Ebola because the majority of the people of Sierra Leone - about 66% - are farmers," he said.

Twelve out of 13 districts in Sierra Leone are now affected by Ebola, although the epicentres are in the Eastern Province near the borders with Liberia and Guinea.

Road blocks manned by police and military are preventing the movement of farmers and labourers as well as the supply of goods.

"We are definitely expecting a devastating effect not only on labour availability and capacity but we are also talking about farms being abandoned by people running away from the epicentres and going to areas that don't have the disease," Mr Sesay added.

Food Shortages

Many shops have been forced to close as part of quarantine measures.

However, the chief co-ordinator for the United Nations Development Programme (UNDP), David McLachlan-Karr, thinks that the road blocks are absolutely crucial to containing the outbreak.

"A robust response to quarantining epicentres of the disease is absolutely necessary," he told the BBC. But he admits agriculture in Sierra Leone has been brought to its knees.

"The stereotypes of Africa as a place of poverty and disease have started to re-emerge again"

Dianna Games Africa@Work

"We are now coming into the planting season which means a lot of agriculture is not happening, so down the line that will create food shortages and pressures on food prices. We are starting to see a rise in inflation and pressure on the national currency as well as a shortage of foreign exchange," he said.

The UNDP has appealed for $18m (£11m) to bolster Sierra Leone's health system while the World Food Programme says the total cost of its emergency operations in Sierra Leone, Guinea and Liberia is $70m.

In Guinea and Liberia the economic predictions may be less catastrophic but they are still worrying. The World Bank said it was expecting GDP growth in Guinea to fall from 4.5% to 3.5%.

Economic growth in Liberia has been revised down due to the outbreak

The Liberian economy had been expected to grow by 5.9% this year but the country's Finance Minister, Amara Konneh, said this was no longer realistic due to a slowdown in the transport and services sectors and the departure of foreign workers because of Ebola.

Mining impact

The world's largest steelmaker ArcelorMittal has seen work disrupted on its iron ore mine expansion project in Yekepa in Liberia, after contractors declared "force majeure" and moved people out of the country.

Simandou, in the forests of eastern Guinea, is Africa's largest iron ore mine and infrastructure project. Vale, the world's biggest iron ore producer, was involved in Simandou until April. It evacuated six international members of staff and put the rest of the workforce in the area on leave.

Rio Tinto, the world's third largest mining company, which owns a share in Simandou, has donated $100,000 to the World Health Organization's work in the area and is also making sanitation equipment available to local people there.

Steelmakers and miners have been hit by the outbreak

A smaller British company, London Mining, has moved out some its non-essential expatriate staff from Sierra Leone, where mining has accounted for much of the country's recent growth. According to the International Monetary Fund, Sierra Leone's output grew by 20% last year; excluding iron ore mining, it grew by 5.5%.

But like Rio Tinto, London Mining has also donated money towards tackling the spread of Ebola, and educating local communities about the virus.

Borders closed

In Sierra Leone, commercial banks have reduced their hours of business by two hours to reduce contact with clients and the country's tourism industry has taken a severe knock - some hotels are empty and are laying off staff.

The closure of borders in West Africa and the suspension of flights are also having a detrimental effect on trade, severely limiting the ability of countries to export and import goods.

Recent examples are the closure of Cameroon's lengthy border with Nigeria and the announcement by Kenya Airways that it is suspending flights to and from Sierra Leone and Liberia.

The outbreak has caused a number of countries to close their borders.

All three West African nations are already poor countries, but the Ebola outbreak could make them even poorer. Sierra Leone and Liberia have both emerged from horrific civil wars and managed to rebuild their economies.

Liberia has been trying to revive its mining sector which before the civil war accounted for more than half its export earnings. But now there are fears that all the good work that has been achieved since those conflicts could be destroyed. There are also concerns that widespread poverty could force people to resort to criminality.

'Fundamentals'

Meanwhile some international investors are nervously watching the Ebola outbreak unfold. Dianna Games, chief executive of

Johannesburg-based consultants Africa@Work, says fears about the virus could damage Africa's economic revival of recent years.

"Ebola has made a dent in the Africa Rising narrative," she told the BBC. "The stereotypes of Africa as a place of poverty and disease have started to re-emerge again."

She thinks Nigeria is the only affected country that has the health system and infrastructure to deal with Ebola. At the moment, all confirmed cases of ebola has been controlled, all of which were linked to the death of one man from Liberia in July.

In the long run, Ms Games believes history will view the 2014 Ebola outbreak as a temporary blip rather than a permanent U-turn in the continent's fortunes.

"The fundamentals pushing this Africa Renaissance are still there," she said.

Ebola: No School Resumption Today In Lagos, 14 Other States

Pupils in at least 15 states in the country will not return to their classrooms today 22 September as directed by the Federal Government of Nigeria.

This is because in most of the states, teachers are insisting that safety measures must be put in place to protect them and their pupils from contracting the deadly Ebola Virus Disease.

In some of the states like Lagos and Ogun, the governments opted not to comply with the September 22 date until necessary Ebola safety kits were put in place in their schools.

And because of the Eid-il-Kabir festival that also falls within this time, rather than open and close the schools again for the festival. Immediately after the festival, the schools will commence academic session on October 8.

This shift in school resumption affected the economy of the private schools' owners in Nigeria as academic session commenced October 8th, 2014.

Ebola: Uzbekistan Bars Nigeria From Wrestling Championships

Uzbekistan, through the world wrestling body FILA, has decided to bar Nigeria and four other African countries from featuring in the 2014 Senior World Wrestling Championships holding in Tashkent, Uzbekistan due to the reported cases of the Ebola Virus Disease in the affected countries.

Sierra Leone, Liberia, Guinea, Congo DR are the other countries barred from the championships and the FILA Congress holding this month in the European country.

The restriction will also deny the African officials from contesting the FILA Bureau elections which hold at the same venue.

Ebola Spoils Business For Sex Workers In Ekiti

…As hawkers now shun Lagos customers over deadly virus

Commercial sex workers, who ply their trade in Ado Ekiti are currently angry. They are angry because the dreaded Ebola disease, which has spread to Lagos, is spoiling business for them.

Checks by Daily Sun in about six brothels in Ado Ekiti revealed that commercial sex workers in the capital city now literally drive away would be customers from Lagos and any prospective client that reveals he is from Lagos.

In the same way, patrons of call girls in Ekiti now ask about the recent movement of any of the prostitutes before choosing who to do business with. This is to find out and avoid those who might have gone to Lagos.

Caf Suspends Matches In Guinea, Liberia & Sierra Leone Due To Ebola Virus

The continental football body says teams from the three countries will play their home games in neutral venues due to the threat of the disease

The Confederation of African Football has ordered the federations of Guinea, Liberia and Sierra Leone to relocate their home matches to neutral venues following the spread of the Ebola virus in those countries.

The national teams of these nations will be participating in the upcoming 2015 Africa Cup of Nations qualifiers set for early September. Their opponents, notably Togo, recently complained to

Caf to move the matches away from those countries due to the threat of the deadly disease, which has devastated regions of Western Africa in recent weeks.

Caf has now ordered fixtures in those countries to be relocated due to the threat of the highly-infectious virus spreading further.

By this development, the home countries will loose all revenues that would have come from ticket sales, adverts etc had the match been played at home.

Catholic Church Moves To Check Ebola Spread

To avert the spread of Ebola Virus Disease (EVD) the Catholic Church may have suspended some aspects of service. These include hand to mouth communion and handshake.

For instance, officiating priests during holy masses in all parishes in the Catholic Archdiocese of Onitsha, will from next Sunday, not give Holy Communion directly with their hands into the mouths of the congregation. This is even as some residents of the Federal Capital Territory (FCT) are coming hard on the Minister, Sen. Bala Mohammed, for allegedly not doing enough in enlightening residents on the deadly disease.

In the Catholic Church, Onitsha, the traditional rite of peace where worshippers shake hands or hug each other during masses will also be skipped henceforth. This procedure was also sidelined in some Catholic churches in Lagos and Mater Misericordiae, Port Harcourt.

'No Handshake, No Sex'

The traditional handshake is no longer a part of salutations in Guinea and Nigeria as people are now really terrified of being infected with Ebola.

An infected person, who may not show symptoms for up to 21 days, can pass on the disease through direct contact.

People also stayed away from sex for the period that ebola lasted in Nigeria.

 "I don't go to any funeral now whether it is an Ebola-related death or not"

Mariam Mansare School teacher.

"I no longer go out of the house just so that I do not have cause to shake people's hands," Mohamed Barry, a 65-year-old retired civil servant, said.

Ebola Patients Buying Survivors' Blood From Black Market – WHO

As hospitals in nations hardest hit by Ebola struggle to keep up, desperate patients are turning to the black market to buy blood from survivors of the virus, the World Health Organization warned.

The deadliest Ebola outbreak in history has killed at least 4000 people in Guinea, Liberia and Sierra Leone — the countries most affected by the virus.

Thousands more are infected and new cases emerge daily globally.

Blood from survivors, referred to as convalescent serum, is said to have antibodies that can fight the deadly virus. Though unproven, it has provided some promise in fighting a disease with no approved drug to treat it.

"Studies suggest blood transfusions from survivors might prevent or treat Ebola virus infection in others, but the results of the studies are still difficult to interpret," the WHO said.

"It is not known whether antibodies in the plasma of survivors are sufficient to treat or prevent the disease. More research is needed."

Convalescent serum has been used to treat patients, including American aid worker Rick Sacra, who is hospitalized in Omaha, Nebraska. He got blood from Kent Brantly, a fellow American who survived Ebola. Both got infected when they were helping patients in Liberia.

But unlike their situation, patients in affected nations are getting blood through improper channels. The illicit trade can lead to the spread of other infections, including HIV and other blood-related ailments.

"We need to work very closely with the affected countries to stem out black market trading of convalescent serum for two reasons," Margaret Chan, WHO's director-general, said this week.

"Because it is in the interest of individuals not to just get convalescent serum without … going through the proper standard and the proper testing because it is important that there may be other infectious vectors that we need to look at."

9 SUPPORT FROM WORLD BODIES

Mark Zuckerberg And Priscilla Chan Donate $25m To Fight Ebola Outbreak

Facebook chief executive Mark Zuckerberg and his wife, Dr Priscilla Chan, are donating $25m to the fight against the worst-ever Ebola outbreak in west Africa.

The money will go to the CDC Foundation, a private, non-profit organization securing donations to help the US Centers for Disease Control and Prevention (CDC) fight the epidemic in west Africa, which has claimed more than 4,000 lives.

"We need to get Ebola under control in the near term so that it doesn't spread further and become a long-term global health crisis that we end up fighting for decades at large scale, like HIV or polio," Zuckerberg said in a post on Facebook. "We believe our grant is the quickest way to empower the CDC and the experts in this field to prevent this outcome."

Zuckerberg's donation more than doubled the contributions toward the Ebola response received by the foundation. Claire Greenwell, a spokeswoman for the foundation, said it has so far received approximately $40m in commitments and donations to help combat the crisis in west Africa. She said the donations will provide critical resources and services needed to improve the situation on the ground in west Africa.

China Announces $32.5m Ebola Aid For Liberia, S'Leone, Guinea

Chinese President Xi Jinping, on Thursday in New Delhi, announced $32.54m aid package for Liberia, Sierra Leone and Guinea to combat the Ebola disease.

He said during his state visit to India that the aid would include cash, food and materials.

Jinping said his country would also provide the World Health Organization with $2m in cash and give the African Union the same amount to fight the disease.

He said the spread of Ebola in West Africa has been a severe challenge for the international community, including China and India.

Jinping said the new package was aimed at helping the three affected West African countries fight the disease and enhance epidemic prevention capability of surrounding countries.

He said it would also support regional organizations concerned to play a leading and coordinating role in fighting the epidemic.

FIFA To Set Up Ebola Treatment Centres In Liberia, Others

President of the International Federation of Football Associations, Sepp Blater, on Saturday said the organization would give full support to three West African countries heavily hit by the Ebola Virus Disease.

According to "Inside Games," an online news provider, Blater made the pledge at FIFA headquarters in Zurich, Switzerland.

The publication stated that the world football's governing body said that the issue would be discussed and agreed upon at its next Finance Committee meeting which would hold in France on Sept. 25.

It said that FIFA had decided to dip into its solidarity fund to help Guinea, Liberia and Sierra Leone, all impoverished countries in West Africa, whose citizens had been afflicted by the Ebola disease.

"FIFA said that the additional financial support would be spent in solidarity with United Nations initiative on the fight against the epidemic.

This announcement, the publication said, came as it emerged that the Antoinette Tubman Stadium in Monrovia, the Liberian capital, was to serve as the site for two large-scale Ebola treatment units.

It stated that the stadium had been identified by the World Health Organisation (WHO) as the safest and most effective location for the units.

It also said that FIFA would cover the costs of any damage to the Monrovia pitch that might be caused by the treatment units.

The publication also quoted Wilfried Lemke, Special Adviser to the Secretary-General of the UN on Sport for Development and Peace as acknowledging that the Ebola outbreak also had tremendous impact on the sport community.

"National authorities, the UN and the world of sport need to work closely together in order to halt the spread of the disease," Lemke said.

FIFA recalled that Nigeria, Sierra Leone and Liberia withdrew from the recent Youth Olympic Games in China because of the Ebola crisis.

EU Releases 140m Euros To Fight Ebola In W'Africa

The European Union has released 140m euros to help countries affected by the deadly Ebola disease in West Africa.

The affected countries are particularly Guinea, Liberia, Sierra Leone and Nigeria. The fund is to help beef up their healthcare systems. The EU made the official announcement on Friday.

In a statement released, the EU said that of the fund, 38m euros would go to strengthening health services and improvement of food security.

In addition, five million euros had been set aside for supplying medical laboratories with essential materials for detecting the Ebola virus and for training local medical staff.

According to the statement, 97.5m euros will support budget operations in Liberia and Sierra Leone in a bid to improve capacity in public services.

It said, "This is with regard to health care and strengthening the macro-economic stability of those countries.

"Specialist teams from the EU project of mobile laboratories arrived in Guinea and Nigeria this week to install mobile laboratories.

"Other specialists will be deployed next week to Liberia with similar equipment."

Japanese Researchers Develop 30-Minute Ebola Test

Japanese researchers said Tuesday they had developed a new method to detect the presence of the Ebola virus in 30 minutes, with technology that could allow doctors to quickly diagnose infection.

Professor Jiro Yasuda and his team at Nagasaki University say their process is also cheaper than the system currently in use in west Africa where the virus has already killed more than 1,500 people. "The new method is simpler than the current one and can be used in countries where expensive testing equipment is not available," Yasuda told AFP by telephone.

"We have yet to receive any questions or requests, but we are pleased to offer the system, which is ready to go," he said.

Yasuda said the team had developed what he called a "primer", which amplifies only those genes specific to the Ebola virus found in a blood sample or other bodily fluid.

Using existing techniques, ribonucleic acid (RNA) -- biological molecules used in the coding of genes -- is extracted from any viruses present in a blood sample.

A health care worker disinfects around the high-risk area at Elwa hospital, run by Medecins Sans Fro ...

This is then used to synthesise the viral DNA, which can be mixed with the primers and then heated to 60-65 degrees Celsius (140-149 Fahrenheit).

If Ebola is present, DNA specific to the virus is amplified in 30 minutes due to the action of the primers. The by-products from the process cause the liquid to become cloudy, providing visual confirmation, Yasuda said.

Currently, a method called polymerase chain reaction, or PCR, is widely used to detect the Ebola virus, which requires doctors to heat and cool samples repeatedly and takes up to two hours.

"The new method only needs a small, battery-powered warmer and the entire system costs just tens of thousands of yen (hundreds of dollars), which developing countries should be able to afford," he added.

The outbreak of the Ebola virus, transmitted through contact with infected bodily fluids, has sparked alarm throughout western Africa and further afield.

UN To Feed One Million In Ebola-Hit Countries

The United Nations is to fly in food aid for up to a million people affected by the Ebola outbreak in West Africa.

According to the World Food Programme, an arm of the UN, the agency is bringing in its own aircraft to make sure food gets through to quarantined areas in Guinea, Liberia and Sierra Leone.

The organization said it would come to the aid of these worst Ebola-hit countries due to the problem of food crisis there.

The WFP Spokesperson, Fabienne Pompey, said, "The restrictions on movement in the most affected areas threatens food security. Commerce is affected; people cannot get to their fields; and prices rise at the markets; so the poorest have trouble feeding themselves."

As a result of the Ebola outbreak, the WFP said it had already started feeding several thousand people in the worst affected areas, including the families of victims who have been quarantined, orphans, old people and hunters hit by the ban on the sale of bush meat.

With several commercial carriers suspending flights to the region because of the epidemic, she said the agency would start a new humanitarian service on Saturday (today) with an aircraft based in Conakry, Guinea which would link the capitals of the three countries.

She said two helicopters would also be brought in to deliver aid to the most isolated areas.

World Bank Pledges $200m To Contain Ebola

The World Bank has pledged $200m to help contain the deadly Ebola virus, with the growing crisis forcing healthcare system in Liberia to shut down out of fear of staff contracting the virus.

The World Bank said on Monday that it would provide up to $200m in emergency assistance to Guinea, Liberia and Sierra Leone to help the West African nations contain the deadly outbreak which has killed 887 since the outbreak began in March this year.

Jim Yong Kim, World Bank president, himself an expert on infectious diseases, said he has been monitoring the spread of the virus and was "deeply saddened" at how it was contributing to the breakdown of "already weak health systems in the three countries".

The funding will help provide medical supplies, pay healthcare staff and take care of other priorities to contain the epidemic and try to prevent future outbreaks, the World Bank said.

The announcement came as health centres in Liberia's capital city of Monrovia shut down because medical personnel became too afraid to turn up to work, the Associated Press news agency reported.

Both Liberia's and Sierra Leone's top Ebola doctors lost their lives to the disease after caring for numerous people.

Healthcare personnel in Liberia say they have not received sufficient support from the government to be able to deal with possible Ebola patients walking through their doors.

"The health workers think that they are not protected, they don't have the requisite material to use as to protect themselves against the Ebola disease, so many of the health workers including physician's assistants, nurses, are staying home," said Amos Richards, a physician's assistant from Monrovia.

Ebola Crisis: WHO To Announce $100m Emergency Response

The head of the World Health Organization and leaders of West African nations affected by the Ebola outbreak are to announce a new $100m (£59m; 75m euro) response plan.

They are meeting in Guinea to launch the initiative to tackle a virus which has claimed 729 lives.

Sierra Leone has declared an emergency after 233 people died there.

Ebola spreads by contact with infected blood, bodily fluids, organs - or contaminated environments.

Initial flu-like symptoms can lead to external haemorrhaging from areas like eyes and gums, and internal bleeding which can lead to organ failure.

Ebola kills up to 90% of those infected, with patients having a better chance of survival if they receive early treatment.

'A new level' WHO Director General Margaret Chan is meeting West African presidents in the Guinean capital Conakry.

"The scale of the Ebola outbreak, and the persistent threat it poses, requires WHO and Guinea, Liberia and Sierra Leone to take the response to a new level, and this will require increased resources, in-country medical expertise, regional preparedness and coordination," she said in a statement released on the WHO website.

"The countries have identified what they need, and WHO is reaching out to the international community to drive the response plan forward."

Key elements of the WHO's new plan are:

- Stopping transmission in the affected countries through "scaling up effective, evidence-based outbreak control measures"

- Preventing the spread of Ebola to "the neighboring at-risk countries through strengthening epidemic preparedness and response measures"

The response builds upon a previous plan that called for several hundred more personnel to be deployed to the region.

The WHO says that the scale of the ongoing outbreak is "unprecedented", with about 1,323 confirmed and suspected cases reported in Guinea, Liberia and Sierra Leone since March 2014.

Liberian President Ellen Johnson Sirleaf has ordered all schools to be closed and put non-essential government workers on leave as part of a series of emergency measures to curtail the Ebola crisis

Office workers in Liberia have been advised to wear gloves as a protective measure to avoid the deadly Ebola virus.

The plan is also expected to highlight the dangers faced by health workers on the front lines of the outbreak, and to call for improving ways to protect them from infection.

'US victim flown to Atlanta' Recently an unnamed US aid worker became infected with the Ebola virus, and was flown for treatment at a high-security ward at Emory University Hospital.

A spokeswoman for the US Centers for Disease Control and Prevention (CDC) said she was not aware of any Ebola patient ever being treated in the US before.

But in a statement the Atlanta hospital said it had an isolation unit which is specially equipped to deal with this kind of infection.

Dr Brantly's condition has deteriorated, but he insisted that a treatment serum be offered to his colleague

Meanwhile an American doctor with Ebola in Liberia has taken a "slight turn for the worse", the Samaritan's Purse aid agency said on Thursday.

Kent Brantly and another American worker, Nancy Writebol, "are in a stable but grave condition", the agency said in a statement.

The statement said that Dr Brantly had been offered experimental serum - using blood from a child whose life he saved - but he had insisted that Ms Writebol should receive it instead.

Health workers, doctors and nurses are a scarce resource in all three countries, and hundreds of international aid workers and more than a hundred WHO staff have already been deployed to support regional response efforts.

WHO says that improving prevention, detecting and reporting suspected cases, referring people infected with the disease for medical care, as well as psychosocial support, are of paramount importance in battling the illness.

The WHO says that more emphasis need to be put on strengthening epidemic preparedness and response measures

The US is sending 50 extra specialists to affected areas.

In other developments:

- President Ellen Johnson-Sirleaf of Liberia - one of the worst hit countries - told the BBC the Ebola outbreak was catastrophic, and more help was needed to contain its spread
- Seychelles have cancelled Saturday's 2015 Africa Cup of Nations qualifier against Sierra Leone because of fears over the Ebola virus
- Nigeria has ordered the temperature screening of passengers arriving from places at risk from Ebola while simultaneously suspending pan-African airline Asky for bringing the first Ebola case to Lagos

In London, the ActionAid charity said that the battle against Ebola was being hampered because of the spiralling price of hand sanitizers.

A spokesman said that the cost of some hygiene products had gone up sevenfold, making them too expensive for many people in the region.

Sierra Leone's President Ernest Bai Koroma announced earlier that the epicentres of the outbreak in the east would be quarantined and he asked the security forces to enforce the measures.

Nigeria Donates $3.5m To Liberia, Others

The Minister of Health, Prof. Onyebuchi Chukwu, on Wednesday said Nigeria had already donated $3.5m as part of its intervention in the affected countries.

Chukwu said the sum was made up of $500,000 to each of the countries and the balance to the common ECOWAS Fund for the disease.

He also said 591 health practitioners had volunteered to join the international force that would go to Liberia, Sierra Leone and Guinea to help in the containment of the Ebola Virus Disease.

He said the volunteers registered with his ministry at three points in Lagos, Abuja and Port-Harcourt.

Chukwu said this while speaking with State House correspondents at the end of the weekly Federal Executive Council meeting presided over by President Goodluck Jonathan.

He said that he had already told a recent meeting of the United Nations General Assembly on EVD of Nigeria's readiness to help the three countries.

He said, "I informed the United Nations General Assembly that the President has already directed the Federal Ministry of Health to train and send health personnel to these three countries in the area of special laboratory work to strengthen capacity in those countries.

"I also informed them that as part of Nigeria's contributions to the international team that will be set up to tackle Ebola Virus Disease in those countries, already Nigeria volunteers from different health professions have been registering with us, willing to join the international force that will go to Liberia, Sierra Leone and Guinea to help out with the containment.

"As of now, 591Nigerians have already registered with us in three registries we opened in Lagos, Abuja Port Harcourt."

The minister however said there were certain conditions to be met before the volunteers would be allowed to leave the country.

He said the first step was for President Goodluck Jonathan to approve their journey and mission and that the volunteers would be properly trained according to Nigeria's standards, which, he said, was fairly high.

Ebola virus disease (EVD)

- Symptoms include high fever, bleeding and central nervous system damage
- Fatality rate can reach 90%
- Incubation period is two to 21 days
- There is no vaccine or cure
- Supportive care such as rehydrating patients who have diarrhoea and vomiting can help recovery
- Fruit bats are considered to be virus' natural host

10 RESOLVING THE ETHICS OF THE EBOLA DILEMMA

A group of ethicists met at the World Health Organization to discuss the wisdom or otherwise of making an experimental drug more widely available to those suffering from Ebola.

Ebola is named after a river in the northern part of the Democratic Republic of Congo. Statistically, it is a relatively trivial disease, killing a few thousand people since its discovery in 1976.

In contrast, malaria and tuberculosis each kill several million people each year. Measles killed 122,000 in 2012. Yet, Ebola has captured the public imagination. We do not know which animal harbours the virus although bats have long been suspected, and this makes prevention and control difficult.

The clinical manifestation is dramatic, with rapid progression from infection to cell death and symptoms that can include bleeding, vomiting and diarrhoea. The fatality rate is high, ranging from 50% to 90%.

Stigma

A common feature of Ebola epidemics is stigma. Sufferers and survivors are often stigmatised by the community, and so too are hospital workers.

"Western medical staff were viewed with suspicion, and sometimes suspected of bringing the disease"

In past outbreaks, some survivors were not welcomed back into their community, some were unable to find work, and some were abandoned by their partners. In the Ugandan outbreak of 2000/2001, the possessions and homes of some survivors were burned.

Volunteers trained by the Red Cross visited villages to dispel myths and persuade them to accept the return of survivors. One survivor of the 1995-1997 outbreaks in Gabon described how people would walk backwards away from him, taxis would not stop and, at roadblocks, police would wave him through for fear of touching his identity card.

Hospitals, often ill-prepared to deal with Ebola, have played a role as amplifiers of epidemics in the past. Many victims since 1976 have been healthcare workers. This gave rise to rumours.

In the 1995 Ebola outbreak in Kikwit, Democratic Republic of Congo, the link between the hospital and those dying of Ebola was such that it generated a popular rumour: doctors were murdering workers who had smuggled diamonds out from the nearby mines.

Hostility

In the Ugandan outbreak, locals believed white people sold the body parts of the victims for profit. Western medical staff were viewed with suspicion, and sometimes suspected of bringing in the disease in.

Every major outbreak of Ebola has been met with local resistance and hostility. In January 2002, an international team of experts fled a village in Mekambo, Gabon, when the villagers threatened them with violence. It is not just the locals who are frightened, but the medical staff too.

The current Ebola outbreak is the biggest yet seen.

Medical historians have documented the cultural disdain for local African customs shown by the colonisers of the early 20th century, for example in the response to the sleeping sickness epidemic that afflicted the Belgian Congo. This sometimes led to revolt on the part of villagers, who were forced to take drugs whose efficacy they doubted and who were touched and prodded in unfamiliar ways.

"A well-known saying in ethics is that 'good ethics starts with good facts'"

Funeral practices have also played a role in spreading the disease, but interfering with these has led to discontent. In past epidemics, locals have simply ignored the recommendations not to bury the dead as before, or not to hunt bush meat.

Some communities have relied on more accessible and familiar traditional healers, and these could spread the disease by cutting the skin or performing other invasive procedures. The health infrastructure in some of the countries afflicted by the disease is poor.

Informed Consent

It is against this complex historical, cultural and social background that the ethicists made a decision. The norms of medical ethics, such as informed consent, may also be different there, and there is a danger in transposing Western norms into different cultures.

A well-known saying in ethics is that "good ethics starts with good facts". Ideally, sitting around that table will be medical historians, anthropologists, clinicians, epidemiologists, logisticians and other specialists. Only then can a nuanced appreciation of the likely risks and benefits be determined.

This will include anticipating what might happen if the drug is introduced and proves ineffective or even harmful, how the media and the local community will react and the consequences of this reaction for victims, healthcare workers, and others, and how the selection process for candidate drugs should take place. Without this input from other disciplines and an understanding of the situation "on the ground", the views of the ethicists may be of limited practical value.

Use Ebola Survivors' Blood To Treat Others - WHO

The blood of patients who recover from Ebola should be used to treat others, the World Health Organization has announced.
West Africa is facing the largest Ebola outbreak in history and more than 4,000 people have died.
A global group of experts have been meeting to assess the experimental therapies that could contain Ebola.

Ebola Treatments: Your Questions Answered

An experimental treatment for Ebola has reportedly shown some signs of success in a US aid worker. What potential treatments for Ebola might be available in the future?

What is the current treatment for Ebola? There is no licensed treatment or vaccine for the Ebola virus. Hospital treatment is based on giving patients intravenous fluids to stop dehydration and antibiotics to fight infections. Strict medical infection control and prompt burial are regarded as the best means of prevention.

What new treatments are being tried for Ebola? A couple of experimental treatments have been used on a compassionate basis. The approach is based on the idea that antibodies against the Ebola virus might help the body fight off the infection. An antibody is a protein produced by the immune system in response to harmful invaders, such as viruses.

What is serum? Serum is the part of the blood that contains antibodies. In past Ebola outbreaks, serum has been taken from people who have survived Ebola but are no longer infectious. Their blood still contains high levels of antibodies against the virus. In one outbreak in 1995 in the Democratic Republic of Congo, seven out of eight patients survived after being treated with serum, according to Prof Tom Solomon, director of the NIHR Health Protection Research Unit in Emerging and Zoonotic infections. Reports suggest that a US aid worker who developed Ebola may have been given serum before being flown home from Africa.

What are monoclonal antibodies? An experimental cocktail of three engineered antibodies against the Ebola virus has been developed. The treatment is not yet licensed as it has not been tested in clinical trials. The antibodies were originally harvested from mice that had been injected with parts of the Ebola virus. They have been adapted to work in the human body and can be manufactured in the tobacco plant.

Experiments on monkeys suggest the antibody cocktail may reduce fatalities when given after exposure to the virus. Two US aid workers have reportedly been given this experimental treatment, known as Zmapp, with "apparently encouraging" signs in one of them, said Prof Solomon.

What other approaches are being tried? There are a couple of prototype vaccines against Ebola, but these are in the very early stages of research in animal models. Nothing is licensed and clinical trials would be very difficult to conduct.

The natural host for the virus is the fruit bat.

The Food and Drug Administration in the US says it is fast-tracking a vaccine that has shown encouraging signs in monkeys for phase 1 trials in September.

This type of trial is the earliest study in humans and aims to make sure that drugs are safe and show some chance of working.

Another area of research is looking into how the Ebola virus triggers severe internal bleeding. The aim would be to boost clotting factors that the body produces naturally to control bleeding.

What are the chances of success? Experts say that pharmaceutical companies are unlikely to invest the huge resources needed to develop new drugs when these would likely be used only occasionally in relatively small numbers of people. They say investment is needed from international agencies to have any realistic chance of success in the future.

How Nigeria Treated Ebola Patients With No Drugs Or Vaccines

How was that possible without vaccines or drugs?

"We needed to understand what was the pathophysiology of the virus. I mean what it causes in the body. Once there is a high fever, the patient starts losing water, fluid and electrolytes because the high fever drains the fluid. Once there is diarrhea and vomiting, the patient loses even more fluid and electrolytes and the patient starts going down. By the time it gets to the stage that the patient is bleeding, you have lost that patient, because he has lost so much. But if you catch them early and as they are losing the fluid, you are replacing the fluid, not necessarily IV, just put a lot of oral dehydration therapy with the patient and be encouraging him to be drinking it, you are replacing the fluid being lost and got them healed without vaccine.

The principal thing is the fluid and electrolyte power which will buy the body sometime. The body itself is a soldier, fighting the virus, but it is at a disadvantage when it is losing fluid and electrolytes. You also need to encourage the patient, since it was not easy to ask somebody to be drinking, considering there is already fear, panic and so on. So, that is why we add the pyscho aspect to encourage the patient. Some patients may benefit from infusion but those are the extreme, if they start bleeding to see if you could win some of them. But the big lesson which I took away from the Ebola importation into the country is that if we are determined as a people, we will achieve results, and where we work as a team, we will achieve results.

Because you could see where the federal and states worked together with a common objective and leaving politics out of it and allowing the professionals to do their job, we were able to achieve results."
Prof. Akin Osibogun said in an interview.

Controlling The Outbreak In Guinea, Liberia, And Sierra Leone

A major challenge is that the three countries are contiguous and in need of independent, coordinated oversight. The case in Nigeria was different because once President Goodluck Jonathan declared a health emergency, he had the authority and resources to direct the entire national effort.

In an attempt to centralize the west African reponse, the current chairman of ECOWAS is the president of Ghana and convening a meeting of west African health ministers together with the director of the Nigerian Center for Disease Control.

In the rest of Africa, Dr. Chukwu suggested that Guinea, Liberia, Sierra Leone (as well as Senegal) could benefit from the expertise of doctors in Uganda and the DRC who have successfully treated Ebola patients. The rest of the world can certainly provide the aid that is starting to grow: emergency mobile hospitals, supplies such as IV fluids and personal protective equipment.

But people in these countries are also voicing a loss of confidence in their own governments as their economies fail and food and clean water are in short supply.

And, particularly with the killing of aid workers in Guinea,the international effort must bolster security to encourage volunteers that they can work safely in what are already extremely demanding conditions.

The Need For Cautious Communication

One challenge in Nigeria was preventing stigmatization of anyone under surveillance as well as Ebola survivors.

"Three terms became part of our lexicon: surveillance, quarantine, and isolation." But these need to be clearly explained, said Dr. Chukwu.

"Surveillance is sort of like house arrest. You don't criminalize them. The person is actually a victim, not a criminal. We monitor their movements, the rest of the family are counseled about what contact can and can't be done. We have contact with them everyday. You can imagine what this effort must've been like when we had 300 in Lagos and over 400 in Port Harcourt."

Only when those under surveillance show symptoms – a fever, whether it ends up being Ebola, yellow fever, or malaria – they are put under quarantine.

"That is the first time we are denying that individual the comfort of his own bed. We put him in separately from the isolation ward from those who are confirmed. If malaria, we discharge them to their doctor to be treated for malaria."

Ebola Fast Facts

(CNN) -- Here's some background information about Ebola, a virus with a high fatality rate that was first identified in Africa in 1976.

Facts:

Ebola hemorrhagic fever is a disease caused by one of five different Ebola viruses. Four of the strains can cause severe illness in humans and animals. The fifth, Reston virus, has caused illness in some animals, but not in humans.

The first human outbreaks occurred in 1976, one in northern Zaire (now Democratic Republic of the Congo) in Central Africa: and the other, in southern Sudan (now South Sudan). The virus is named after the Ebola River, where the virus was first recognized in 1976, according to the Centers for Disease Control and Prevention.

Ebola is extremely infectious but not extremely contagious. It is infectious, because an infinitesimally small amount can cause illness. Laboratory experiments on nonhuman primates suggest that even a single virus may be enough to trigger a fatal infection.

Instead, Ebola could be considered moderately contagious, because the virus is not transmitted through the air. The most contagious diseases, such as measles or influenza, virus particles are airborne.

Humans can be infected by other humans if they come in contact with body fluids from an infected person or contaminated objects from infected persons. Humans can also be exposed to the virus, for example, by butchering infected animals.

While the exact reservoir of Ebola viruses is still unknown, researchers believe the most likely natural hosts are fruit bats.

Symptoms of Ebola typically include: weakness, fever, aches, diarrhoea, vomiting and stomach pain. Additional experiences include rash, red eyes, chest pain, throat soreness, difficulty breathing or swallowing and bleeding (including internal).

Typically, symptoms appear 8-10 days after exposure to the virus, but the incubation period can span two to 21 days.

Unprotected health care workers are susceptible to infection because of their close contact with patients during treatment.

Ebola is not transmissible if someone is asymptomatic or once someone has recovered from it. However, the virus has been found in semen for up to three months.

Deadly human Ebola outbreaks have been confirmed in the following countries: Democratic Republic of the Congo (DRC), Gabon, South Sudan, Ivory Coast, Uganda, Republic of the Congo (ROC),Guinea and Liberia.

According to the World Health Organization, "there is no specific treatment or vaccine," and the fatality rate can be up to 90%. Patients are given supportive care, which includes providing fluids and electrolytes and food.

There are five subspecies of the Ebola virus: Zaire ebolavirus (EBOV), Bundibugyo ebolavirus (BDBV), Sudan ebolavirus (SUDV), Taï Forest ebolavirus (TAFV) and Reston ebolavirus (RESTV)

2014 West Africa Outbreak:

(Full historical timeline at bottom)

Cases listed below include confirmed, ***probable*** or suspected cases of Ebola as of September 23, 2014 and beyond(World Health Organization and CDC):

Guinea - 1074 cases, 648 deaths

Liberia - 3458 cases, 1830 deaths

Nigeria - 20 cases, 8 deaths

Senegal - 1 case, 0 deaths

Sierra Leone - 2021 cases, 605 deaths

March 25, 2014 - The CDC issues its initial announcement on an outbreak in Guinea, and reports of cases in Liberia and Sierra Leone. "In Guinea, a total of 86 suspected cases, including 59 deaths (case fatality ratio: 68.5%), had been reported as of March 24, 2014.

Preliminary results from the Pasteur Institute in Lyon, France suggest Zaire ebolavirus as the causative agent."

April 16, 2014 - The New England Journal of Medicine publishes a report, speculating that the current outbreak's Patient Zero was a two-year-old from Guinea. The child died on December 6, 2013, followed by his mother, sister and grandmother over the next month.

July 2014 - Patrick Sawyer, a top government official in the Liberian Ministry of Finance, dies at a local Nigerian hospital. He is the first American to die in what officials are calling "deadliest Ebola outbreak in history."

July 2014 – Nancy Writebol, an American aid worker in Liberia, tests positive for Ebola. According to Samaritan's Purse, Writebol is infected while treating Ebola patients in Liberia.

July 26, 2014 – Kent Brantly,medical director for Samaritan Purse's Ebola Consolidated Case Management Center in Liberia, is infected with the virus. According to Samaritan's Purse, Brantly is infected while treating Ebola patients.

July 29, 2014 - According to Doctors Without Borders, Dr. Sheik Humarr Khan who was overseeing Ebola treatment at Kenema Government Hospital in Sierra Leone dies from complications of the disease..

July 30, 2014 – The Peace Corps announces it is removing its volunteers from Liberia, Sierra Leone and Guinea.

July 31, 2014 – CDC raises its warning to Level 3. It warns U.S. residents to avoid "nonessential travel" to Sierra Leone, Guinea, and Liberia.

August 2, 2014 – A specially equipped medical plane carrying Ebola patient Dr. Kent Brantly lands at Dobbins Air Reserve Base in Marietta, Georgia. He is then driven by ambulance to Emory University Hospital in Atlanta.

August 4, 2014 - CNN reports that that top secret, experimental vials of the drug, "ZMapp" were flown into Liberia last week in a last-ditch effort to save Brantly and Writebol, according to a source familiar with details of the treatment. Doctors report "significant improvement."

August 6, 2014 - Nancy Writebol arrives at Emory in Atlanta for treatment.

August 8, 2014 - Experts at the World Health Organization declare the Ebola epidemic ravaging West Africa an international health emergency that requires a coordinated global approach, describing it as the worst outbreak in the four-decade history of tracking the disease.

August 19, 2014 - Liberia's President Ellen Johnson Sirleaf declares a nationwide curfew beginning August 20 and orders two communities to be completely quarantined, with no movement in or out of the areas.

August 21, 2014 - Dr. Kent Brantly is discharged from Emory University Hospital. It is also announced that Nancy Writebol had been released on Tuesday, August 19. The releases come after Emory staff are confident Brantly and Wrtebol pose "no public health threat."

September 6, 2014 - The government of Sierra Leone announces plans for a nationwide lockdown from September 19-21, in order to stop the spread of Ebola. The lockdown is being billed as a predominantly social campaign rather than a medical one, in which volunteers will go door-to-door to talk to people.

September 16, 2014 – President Barack Obama calls the efforts to combat the Ebola outbreak centered in West Africa "the largest international response in the history of the CDC." Speaking from the CDC headquarters in Atlanta, Obama adds that "faced with this outbreak, the world is looking to" the United States to lead international efforts to combat the virus. He says the United States is ready to take on that leadership role.

September 30, 2014 - Dr. Thomas Frieden, director of the CDC, announces the first diagnosed case of Ebola in the United States. The person has been hospitalized and isolated at Texas Health Presbyterian Hospital in Dallas, Texas, since September 28.

October 1, 2014 - Liberian government officials release the name of the first diagnosed case of Ebola in the United States: Thomas Eric Duncan.

October 8, 2014 - Thomas Eric Duncan dies.

October 14, 2014 – UN health worker dies in Germany.

October 20, 2014 – WHO declares end of Ebola outbreak in Nigeria.

October 20, 2014 – Emory's third Ebola patient is discharged.

October 21, 2014 - Ashoka Mukpo, an American freelance television cameraman working for NBC News in Liberia, declared free of Ebola.

October 23, 2014 - Doctor diagnosed positive for Ebola in New York.

Timeline:

*Includes outbreaks resulting in more than 100 deaths or special cases.

1976 - First recognition of the EBOV disease is in Zaire (now Democratic Republic of the Congo). The outbreak has 318 reported human cases, leading to 280 deaths. An SUDV outbreak also occurs in Sudan (now South Sudan), which incurs 284 cases and 151 deaths.

1989 - In Reston, Virginia, macaque monkeys imported from the Philippines are found to be infected with the Ebola virus (later named the Ebola-Reston virus).

1990 - In Texas and Virginia quarantine facilities, four humans develop Ebola antibodies after contact with monkeys imported from the Philippines. None of the humans has symptoms.

1995 - An outbreak in Democratic Republic of the Congo (formerly Zaire) leads to 315 reported cases and at least 250 deaths.

2000-2001 - A Ugandan outbreak (SUDV) results in 425 human cases and 224 deaths.

2001-2002 - An EBOV outbreak occurs on the border of Gabon and Republic of the Congo (ROC), which results in 53 deaths on the Gabon side and at least 43 deaths on the Republic of the Congo side.

December 2002-April 2003 - An EBOV outbreak in Republic of the Congo results in 143 reported cases and 128 deaths.

2007 - An EBOV outbreak occurs in the Democratic Republic of the Congo (DRC), 187 of the 264 cases reported result in death. In late 2007, an outbreak in Uganda leads to 37 deaths. 149 cases were reported.

November 2008 - The Ebola-Reston virus (RESTV) is detected in five humans in the Philippines. They are workers on a pig farm and slaughterhouse and suffer no symptoms. This is the first known occurrence of the Reston virus in pigs.

August 26, 2014 - The Ministry of Health in the Democratic Republic of the Congo notifies the World Health Organization of an Ebola outbreak in the country. It is the seventh outbreak in the country since 1976, when the virus was first identified near the Ebola river. The outbreak is not related to the ongoing outbreak in Guinea, Liberia, Nigeria and Sierra Leone. As of September 24, 70 cases and 42 deaths have been reported in the Democratic Republic of the Congo.

Ebola Outbreak: Six Surprising Numbers

1.7

people infected by each Ebola sufferer in Liberia

The figure of 1.7 means that, on average, every 10 people infected with Ebola in Liberia will have passed the disease on to 17 others. This figure is known as a basic reproduction number. It is used to measure the rate at which an epidemic spreads through a susceptible population. The number fluctuates as scientists keep monitoring new cases.

By comparison, measles - a highly contagious disease - can have a reproduction number of between 12 and 17.

Figure from European Centre for Disease Prevention and Control

Line.

19,980

burial kits needed

The bodies of Ebola victims remain infectious after death. Safe burials are key to checking the spread of the disease.

Figure from UN Office for the Co-ordination of Humanitarian Affairs (Ocha)

line

1 in 50

Liberian health workers infected

Ebola is transmitted through patients' body fluids, leaving health workers particularly vulnerable to the disease. Where medics have lacked adequate protection, their rate of infection has been higher.

Figure from Ocha

line

$61.48

cost of a full protective suit

The suit must be worn by medical personnel to protect against infection. It includes a protective mask, goggles, apron, gloves and rubber boots.

Figure from Medecins Sans Frontieres

line

5,060

mobile phones needed

The medical teams now being sent to the affected countries need mobile phones to pass on vital information about how the disease is spreading, especially in remote areas.

Figure from Ocha

line

90 days

without sex for survivors of Ebola

The Ebola virus can remain present in semen for a long time. Experts say it is best for men who are recovering from the disease to avoid sex altogether - or make sure they use a condom - for 90 days.

Figure from Peter Piot, of the London School of Hygiene and Tropical Medicine, who discovered Ebola in 1976.

Ebola Survivors' Testimonies

Dr. Ada Igonoh Shares Her Story

Although more than 4,447 victims have died in the largest Ebola outbreak in history, one woman's story of survival could be a sign of hope for those that are still battling the illness.

Dr. Ada Igonoh contracted Ebola in Nigeria after treating Patrick Sawyer, an American who died of the disease in July, the head of the Ebola Emergency Operation Center confirmed to HuffPost Live. In an interview on Monday, Igonoh recalled how she caught the virus and her road to recovery in the confines of an isolation center in Nigeria.

"At the time when I contracted the virus, it must have been when I touched [Sawyer's] intravenous fluid bag, one of the nights I was attending to him," she told host Alyona Minoyski. "About a week after the contact with him ... it was confirmed that I had Ebola."

After Igonoh's diagnosis, she was rushed to the Emergency Operation Center's isolation area for treatment.

"I had some infections, so I had to be treated with antibiotics to treat the infection. After about a week of staying in the isolation ward, I started to feel much better," she said. "The symptoms, mainly fever, diarrhea and vomiting with associated joint aches and pains, actually started to resolve at that time."

After being treated with Paracetamol and oral rehydration salts, Igonoh's symptoms slowly started to subside. Fourteen days later, she was declared "virus free" and released from the ward.

While the average fatality rate for Ebola is around 70 percent, according to the World Health Organization, Igonoh is optimistic about the possibilities for treatment and survival.

"Even [though] there is no known cure for Ebola, or no known vaccine for Ebola, usually people are treated symptomatically," Igonoh said. "And once the symptoms can be treated and dehydration aggressively treated, or prevented, the possibility of living is quite high."

I Caught Ebola In Guinea And Survived

One survivor, who asked not to be named, told the BBC his story.

Testimony:

The symptoms started with headaches, diarrhoea, pains in my back and vomiting.

"None of us could sleep - we thought we would never make it to the morning"

The first doctor I saw at a village health centre said it was malaria - it was only when I was brought to a special unit at the hospital in [the capital] Conakry that I was told I had the Ebola virus.

I felt really depressed - I had heard about Ebola so when the doctors told me, I was very scared.

I tried to be positive - I was thinking about death, but deep inside I thought my time had not come yet and I would get over it. That's how I overcame the pain and the fear.

Doctors from the charity Medecins Sans Frontiers (MSF) were here to comfort me and give their moral support. I tried to stay positive although I was scared when I saw my relatives dying in front of me.

There was a moment when I thought I might die when I lost two of my uncles and their bodies were taken away.

On that night none of us could sleep - we thought we would never make it to the morning.

Some doctors from MSF came to collect and wrap the bodies and sterilize the area. It all happened in front of us.

A short while after I was admitted to the hospital for treatment I started feeling better, step by step.

'Shook my hands'

At first I was scared to eat as I thought I would be sick but after a while I took a few drops of water and realised it was OK and the diarrhoea gradually stopped as well.

www.ingramcontent.com/pod-product-compliance
Lightning Source LLC
Chambersburg PA
CBHW070604290526
45790CB00002B/769